MEDICINE, MISTAKES, AND THE REPTILIAN BRAIN

The NewMind Response™ to Better Decisions

MEDICINE, MISTAKES, AND THE REPTILIAN BRAIN

The NewMind Response™ to Better Decisions

by

Dr. John Mary Meagher

Meagher, John M.
    Medicine, Mistakes and the Reptilian Brain / John Mary Meagher.

ISBN 978-1470177324
    I. Title.

Designed by Chris Tucker

Printed and bound in Canada

AHYMSA PUBLISHING
120 Branch Street
Moncton, NB, E1A 4Y1
Canada

…and we must acknowledge, as it seems to me, that man with all his noble qualities, with sympathy which feels for the most debased, with benevolence which extends not only to other men but to the humblest living creature, with his godlike intellect which has penetrated into the movements and constitution of the solar system with all these exalted powers Man still bears in his bodily frame the indelible stamp of his lowly origin.
-Charles Darwin.

Theorem of Attribution:
To err is human, the reptilian part of the human.
-John Mary Meagher

The real cycle you're working on is a cycle called yourself.
…Working on a motorcycle, working well, caring, is to become part of a process, to achieve an inner peace of mind.
-Robert Pirsig

For Bridget Bernadette

PREFACE

- Betsy Lehman ... died from an overdose during chemotherapy.
- Willie King had the wrong leg amputated.
- Ben Kolb was eight years old when he died during "minor" surgery due to a drug mixup.[1]

This is the stark opening of the Institute of Medicine's 2002 Report on the Quality of Health Care entitled "To Err is Human."

The Institute of Medicine concludes: "Given current knowledge about the magnitude of the problem, the committee believes it would be irresponsible to expect anything less than a 50 percent reduction in errors over five years."[2]

About four years prior to the Institute's report, one of my mistakes jolted me to research the nature of error. I searched for the causes of my errors in the system, the staff, and the patients. But I found that the cause was myself. I also found that non-ownership of error only leads through a desert of aimlessness, where one can find no bearing from which to improve. Error admitted, on the other hand, can bring one to an oasis of meaning and self-knowledge, a starting point from which to improve one's work.[3]

Approximately 80% of aviation mishaps and errors are due to human factors. The same is true for medical errors. These human factors are expressions of our reptilian brain, which follows an agenda of self-interest. (We can divide the human brain into two control centers, the old [reptilian] and the new. The reptilian brain screens and reacts to signs of threat, food, mating possibilities and fatigue. The new brain, on the other hand, discerns, ponders, postpones, tests and responds to problems. We can toggle unknowingly from the new center to the old one). The physician's new brain is the repository of the patient's well-being. If we can mitigate the reptilian brain's influences and enhance the new brain's influences, we will make fewer mistakes. This dual activity I call the NewMind Response™.

It is as easy to recognize reptilian brain expressions in others as it is difficult to spot them in ourselves. Robbie Burns recognized this difficulty when seeing lice on a lady's hat, he remarked:

> "O would some Power the gift give us
> To see ourselves as others see us!
> It would from many a blunder free us."

And to free us from many a blunder is the sole aim and hope of this book.

-Dr. John Mary Meagher

P.S. Though this book is set in the hospital, the workshop of my errors and research, the non-medical reader should also benefit, because the reptilian brain can corrupt judgment and compromise work, spoil exchanges between partners and between parents and children. Medical jargon is explained in the References and Notes section.

TABLE OF CONTENTS

Acknowledgments   **131**

References and Notes   **133**

INTRODUCTION

MY ERROR, MY POST-MORTEM
Can one separate the diagnostician from the misdiagnosis?

After many years of medical practice, I awoke one night replaying an incident from my youth. "Seamus and John, check the fire in the field," our father had ordered my brother and me. I was 10 then. I ran to the ditch that bordered the field, saw no smoke from the bundle of sticks in the field and ran back to my father. "The fire is dead." I declared. Seamus, on the other hand, went around through the gate to the fire and kicked it to make sure that it was quenched. It was still smoldering. "That fire could have burned the house down," my father chastised me. "If you are going to do a job, do it with your whole being, John. You'll have to do better, otherwise you'll end up a slacker."

I dream such dreams of self-criticism whenever I make a major blunder in the emergency department. Who was it this time? Ah, yes. It was the 83-year-old man, who was triaged to the 12th bed of the acute part of the emergency department. Let's rename him, Mr. Weston. What happened to him? I leapt out of bed at two o'clock in the morning, twelve hours after I had seen him. The day before, the patient's general practitioner had called me. "He's just constipated. His family is bugging me about him. I've a full office, could you see him for me? Give me a call about him." I had agreed to see him.

As I sat on the edge of my bed, I recalled the man lying on a stretcher, flanked by two concerned women, a suitcase beside them, a sure sign that the relatives believe the patient should be admitted to the hospital.

I had asked the two women to wait in the waiting room, and I would talk to them after I had seen the patient. Mr. Weston told me that he had been constipated for one week and was having pain in his lower abdomen. Straight away, I palpated his abdomen. His lower abdomen was distended and mildly tender, and his upper abdomen was soft. Rectal examination showed normal stool that was negative for occult blood. I ordered the usual blood and X-ray studies and spoke to his two friends in fur coats and expensive-looking jewelry. They told me that his family physician had reassured them that he would be admitted to the hospital because he was so weak.

I eased back in my bed and asked myself, "How weak was he?" I sensed myself blush because hours earlier I had not asked, "What change have you seen in him? How weak was he?" I had not asked him to get up and walk, or measured his blood pressure upon standing. Rather, I had bristled at his two friends or relatives. (I now realize that my bristling was a sign that my intellectual esteem had been impugned by these two advocates.) "The family physician may have told you, but he did not tell me," I rallied. "If you want to wait an hour or two, I will have the results of the tests, and then I will have a better idea of whether he will be admitted or not."

Un cowed, one of his friends countered, "Did he have a stroke?" "No." I replied, "He can move all limbs." Again, I had been prompted a second time to explore his weakness. But I was in a hurry to see other patients and walked away. I did not see them again.

Lying back in bed I could feel my blood rush up my neck. His blood [4] reports were normal except for the B.U.N. which was slightly elevated. The consultant radiologist had told me that my patient's acute abdominal series "was full of shit." I had then ordered an enema and planned to admit him. Later, his nurse, who had given him the enema, told me that it had not worked. "All quiet on the cistern front," I laughed, but his nurse countered as an empowered advocate should: "I know this man, he is an able chess-player, and he is not himself." I had rejected this third prompt to explore why he was different from his usual self.

From my bed, I telephoned the hospital, and his attending nurse told me. "He is dead. He arrested and they could not save him." I put the tele- phone down. A flood of emotions overwhelmed me. Only hours since I had admitted him. Constipation had not killed him. What a slacker I was. I wished then that they would strip me of my medical license.

What was the medical reason for his death? I had no idea. A stroke? Silent myocardial infarction? Though I was free the following day, I re- turned to the hospital to find the pathologist's answer.

As I was driving to the hospital, I mulled over my inattention to my patient. Then I noticed that I had driven through the flashing amber lights of a pedestrian crossing. It was signaling for two young pedestri- ans who were crossing. I did not see that another car had already stopped, and I nearly ran down two junior high students. I should pay attention to what I am doing. When driving the car I should focus on the road, and when diagnosing a patient I should focus on that. Inat- tention, I thought, is transient blindness and transient deafness. Inat- tention is easy. One step toward it and one has already arrived, arrived at transient blindness and transient deafness. Attention, on the other hand, is a bucking bronco, difficult to ride for more than a few seconds. On the way to the hospital I strove to concentrate on the road, the traffic and the stop signs, but I found that I was fervently praying that his diagnosis was something that had occurred after I had seen him, like a pulmonary embolism, a sub-arachnoid haemorrhage. "Please," I thought, "let it be some illness that would not inculpate me."

My prayers were not answered. The pathologist pronounced, "Volvulus. Volvulus and no urine in the bladder." Volvulus is the rota- tion of a segment of bowel about its mesenteric axis obstructing its lumen and blood supply. I showed three other radiologists his X-rays and they all agreed on volvulus. Alas (I used another four-lettered Anglo-Saxon word), I had been given a wrong turn by the radiologist.

I sat in one of the confessional-like booths of Medical Records, and stared at the patient's chart. Now I had plenty of time to ponder the patient's case. Why did I not bring the same attention when he was alive? His vital signs[5] jumped off the page at me. They were abnormal: blood pressure 90/50, pulse /min. They indicated that he was in shock and explained his weakness. How could I blame the medical system, though it has been described as having sharp ends?[6] What brutish system could blind me to abnormal vital signs written clearly on a page? Yet the fox will condemn the trap, never itself. I saw the vital signs now because I was both humbled and puzzled.

I read the nurses' notes. His attending nurse on the floor had told his family physician that the patient's blood pressure had dropped, and an hour later she informed him that the patient had not produced urine in the last ten hours. His family physician had hugged the horizontal. This is an apathy reminiscent of Sir Thomas Huxley's remark, "Nothin is too good for the patient, provided it doesn't involve any extra effort on my part."

Another doctor entered the Medical Records' Room. I could not bring myself to utter the basic salutation of one being to another. I imagined my recent error emitted some loathsome aura. I was in a free fall to the inescapable conclusion that I was a space-occupying lesion of negligence which had metastasized to others before and now to this patient with the volvulus. What was this negligence? Psychologists might call it a framing error.[7] This term felt euphemistic[8] to me; it understated both my clear ownership and the depth of the guilt I commanded for this mortal error.

Is there a way to atone in medicine? The injury is sometimes irreparable: the scarred heart muscle of a missed heart attack, cerebral palsy from fetal anoxia, and in this case, a life. How could one atone for that? Also, I knew of no propitiation, no penance to mitigate the wrong.[9]

My previous medical errors, some obstetrical, some cardiac, returned like forgotten creditors to attest my medical bankruptcy. All my well intentioned years of medical care and successes could not balance these other debts. I sank into that underworld where hope, confidence, and collegiality are lost, and I am banished like a leper to meander through my labyrinth of shame, anguish, fear, and unalloyed worthless- ness, at the core of which lies the heart of darkness.[10]

Can performing a post-mortem on error be helpful? Am I a recidivist to inattention and to guessing? A slacker? Is the child always father to the man? Celebrated sportsman Bobby Jones Jr. valued the post-mortem of error: "I never learned from my successes, only learned from my drabbings." Pasteur said that discovery favored the prepared mind. A diagnosis, also a discovery, must favor the prepared mind. Yet medical schools have been inattentive to preparing the mind to meet the patient, inattentive to errors, inattentive to attention, inattentive to inattention and inattentive to the study of the self, which is to be inattentive to the minefield within.

From this crisis of pulsating shame and crowding loneliness, I resolved to improve. Regret without the resolve to improve is insincere, a devil's contrition. I have striven to learn about error, which is to learn about myself. For one can no more separate the diagnostician from the misdiagnosis than the slacker from the burned down house.[11]

How could one improve? Could one improve at all? I began with a bald, banal but irrefutable claim of Cicero's, "the nature of man is to err." What is this nature? The accounts of 19 doctors' errors in the first chapter will help us understand.

Part I: REDUCING ERROR

Chapter 1

Nineteen Doctors' Errors and the Theorem of Attribution of Error to the Reptilian Brain

"...errors tend to take a surprisingly limited number of forms."
-James Reason [12]

The accounts of 19 physicians recounting their own mistakes reveal a surprisingly limited number of attitudes. In "Perceived Causes of Family Physicians' Errors,"[13] 14 family physicians give verbatim ac- counts of their "most memorable" errors. The other five accounts are by internists from the article, "The Heart of Darkness."[14] I place the accounts in italics, the salient attitudes in bold font and my comments in regular font.

1. *I was in a hurry and I just didn't stop to think about all the possibilities. I mean I know about (name of the disease), they teach that in medical school and I knew about it....But I just didn't even think about it.....But I didn't even think about it. I was just in a hurry, you know, in a hurry to get to the next (patient).* **HASTE**

2. *At that point, I was still in training and I wasn't completely competent when it came to technical things, I was fatigued, I was fearful of looking as incompetent as I*

was, so that I didn't feel that I could call on the people that I really needed to help me. I wasn't supposed to be calling. That was a sign that you were a wuss'. **EGOISM and FATIGUE.** Egoism occurs when concern about one's self-esteem preempts the patient's well-being.

3. Since I've had time to reflect on this, I probably was busy thinking of an upcoming trip that we always take and I didn't remember to... Again a lack of concentration on my part and probably a little bit of preoccupation getting this office set up for (my absence). **HASTE and CONVENIENCE**[15]

4. Because to convince these guys to drive an hour and a half to go to (name of city) to get a CT scan and then (it would) be midnight and then try to convince the physician that I thought this person needed a CT scan... uh (shakes head).... You know, they'd say, "Yeah, right, doc." **EGOISM and possibly CONVENIENCE**

5. And I can see, looking back... where you try and make it fit something less than it is to justify your course of action and plan at the time. I can see all those other pressures where everybody wants to shut down the clinic. It's been a long day, get home, get out. Do I really want to go up and do all this stuff? Do I want to have the (consultant) see him, do I want to do the blood count, and the (procedure) and mess with trying to get an IV started and all those other things that very quickly go through your mind, and you say, "Well, I don't think the patient is that sick." **CONVENIENCE, HASTE and EGOISM.**

6. All of a sudden, they were just suddenly concerned,
7. to the point where they were really irritating me. Like, "Did you check this, did you check this?" And the mother was in between me and the patient and wouldn't get out of the way so I could look at the patient. She wasn't doing this on purpose, but I was really getting angry. I examined her again, I don't find anything specific. And I'm really angry now. And by this time I'm not listening, I'm not making the right decisions, I'm saying, "'Absolutely not...'" **IRRITABILITY and EMPHATIC EXPRESSION**

7. And she was very obnoxious to my nurse (who said), 'This lady's really not a very nice lady.' And so my nurse kind of gives me a little preview, you know,

2

so I was ready to go in there and thinking ... (But) she wasn't obnoxious to me. She was actually kind of nice (tentative tone of voice). But then she got up off the exam table, she had a hundred questions. She stood there and they were these bizarre questions, and (with) each question I got more and more irritated.

LABELING and IRRITABILITY By labeling, I mean a non professional and or pejorative judgment that is frequently kindled by dislike or inconvenience.

8. *And I was thinking, does this guy have a (malignancy) or something, but of course, being a friend, I didn't want him to have anything bad so once I did that (normal study), I just kind of put it out of my mind.... because I just didn't want him to be sick.* **LABELING** Here the labeling is due to liking the patient. Pasteur warned, "The greatest disorder of the mind is to allow the will to direct belief."

9. *And I talked to him about the fact that he should see a cardiologist and he wasn't....In retrospect I probably should have pushed him to see him that he felt, "Ahh, it'll be fine," and so I didn't push it really that much, and (sigh) I wasn't aggressive enough to push him to see the cardiologist immediately.* **APATHY**

10. *But in the course of the exam I found what I thought was a (mass) on the left, and I evaluated him with an imaging study and it turned out normal. So I just kind of put it out of my mind.* I detected no hazardous attitude in this account.

11. *I guess his age, relatively young, the thought of (cancer) didn't even raise... I didn't think of it. I flat out didn't think of (the) connection of bone pain secondary to (cancer), I just didn't mainly because he was younger, and he wasn't aggressive... and it's not his fault, it's mine.* **LABELING.** In labeling the patient as young, the physician dismissed the possibility of serious pathology. Labeling can be treacherous, discouraging due diligence and care.

The last three accounts (12, 13, & 14) from the Ely group describe forms of panic. Here the throbbing reptilian brain switches off any new brain input.

12. *He kept complaining, "My chest, it hurts, it hurts, it hurts."... I always*

3

felt that I over-treated I just think overreaction to the history, because I could still see him lying there, you know (demonstrates by clutching chest). He kept saying, "So do something! Do something!" You feel like you have to do something And I thought, (expletive deleted), he's gonna die from (name of disease), so you start to treat him. **IMPULSIVITY**

13. *...inexperienced, didn't know exactly what to do and panicked I guess you'd say. And he ultimately died, because I didn't know what to do with him. So I...needless to say, I looked up the treatment for (name of disease), and I still remember it all very well.* Though panic is described here, it is secondary to incompetence. Incompetence is more an inability than an attitude.

14. *They arrived and this guy was in terrible shape. He was bleeding like gangbusters. Here's where I screwed up. I forgot all the basic training about stabilizing the patient. I got so excited about all the horrible injuries, that I didn't tend to business.* **IMPULSIVITY**

15. *....the physician was in a hurry because his partner's patient had been worked into his schedule on a busy Friday afternoon.* **HASTE and CONVENIENCE**

16. *Another physician felt that his negligence in not checking for allergies to a medication had been due to fatigue.* **FATIGUE**

17. *One physician felt that pride had prevented him from readmitting a patient he had previously discharged.* **EGOISM**

18. *Another doctor shared the perception that being chronically busy because of a large patient load had led him to be lax in supervising subordinates.* **APATHY and HASTE**

19. *Some physicians believed that the probability of a serious mistake increased with age and experience...(because) you have constraints practicing, seeing a lot of people in a short space of time, having to make very quick judgments that do not appreciate certain data, having to take short cuts.* **HASTE**

These physicians attribute their errors to: Haste, Impulsivity, Fatigue, Egoism, Stress, Convenience, Irritability, Apathy, and Labeling. These can be reduced to the three major causes of errors: Haste, Egoism and Apathy.

Convenience, Stress, Irritability, Emphatic Expression and Impulsivity are sometimes associated with Haste.

Labeling, Fatigue, Stress, Convenience and Irritability can be associated with Apathy.

Finally, Irritability, Convenience, Empathic Expression and Labeling are sometimes associated with Egoism.

Throughout my research, medical authorities defer to and quote from the commercial aviation industry. Its safety record is stellar. For every million commercial airplane departures there are 1.3 hull damages. They have found that the human factor contributes to about 80% of mishaps and errors. The industry has created courses for crews, called Crew Resource Management (CRM). One of the course objectives is: "… to enhance participants' abilities to utilize their most valuable resource-THEMSELVES."[16]

The aviation industry has identified six hazardous attitudes in the cockpit.[17] They are:

IMPULSIVITY: "Do something quickly." When fire started in one engine a British Midland crew turned off the fuel to the functioning engine instead of the malfunctioning one. Eight percent of the physicians in the Ely group felt that panic led to an inadequate performance in a crisis.

PRESSING ATTITUDE: "Let's hurry and get this thing done so we can go home." In the Ely group, 57% of physicians felt hurried. Five (Nos. 1, 2, 5, 15 & 19) of the verbatim accounts reflect pressing attitudes.

MACHOISM: "I can do it." They prove themselves by taking risks and by trying to impress others. It is called the air show syndrome: "I'm going to look so good." Two (2, & 17) verbatim accounts demonstrate machoism. Also 23% of the physicians in the Ely group claimed that they had reached beyond their capabilities.

ANTI-AUTHORITY: "Don't tell me." This attitude of "don't tell me" was present in No.6 of the verbatim accounts. I resented the relatives and the nurse of my patient, who had a volvulus, when they challenged me.

INVULNERABILITY: "It won't happen to me." One may feel invulnerable working in an after-hours clinic where secretaries defer serious problems to emergency departments and accept low-acuity cases. Occasionally a serious problem can filter through. There's a joker in the pack. I recall working in an after-hours clinic one evening when I saw a seven-year-old girl who had had a cough for two days. I noticed that her nostrils were flaring and her respiratory rate was 50 per minute. She died two days later. Where one sees a patient is no reflection on the gravity of their problems.

RESIGNATION: "What's the use?" They do not see themselves as making a great deal of difference in what happens. Sometimes, such individuals will even go along with unreasonable requests just to be a "nice guy". Verbatim accounts (4 & 5) show the pressures to comply with the prevailing culture.

These six hazardous attitudes can also be grouped into the same three causes of error:

Impulsivity and Pressing Attitude: to Haste;
Machoism and Anti-Authority: to Egoism;
Invulnerability and Resignation: to Apathy.

Haste, Egoism, and Apathy[18] are expressions of our evolutionary old brain (archi-cortex). Osler noted the power of the older brain to err: "In the first place, in the physician or surgeon no quality takes rank with imperturbability... Even under the most serious circumstances, the physician or surgeon who... shows in his face the slightest alteration, expressive anxiety or fear, has not his *medullary centres* under the highest control, and is liable to disaster at any moment"(italics mine).

Our brain can be divided into two parts, the old brain (archi-cortex or reptilian) and the new brain (neo-cortex) (Figure 1).The older brain corresponds to the reptilian brain, which consists of the brain stem and the limbic system.[19]

To see how the old brain expresses itself, observe the reptile.

For its survival, the reptile processes stimuli in nanoseconds. Stimuli are reflexively labeled friend, foe or food, and it reacts instantly and emphatically. **(IMPULSIVITY, HASTE)**

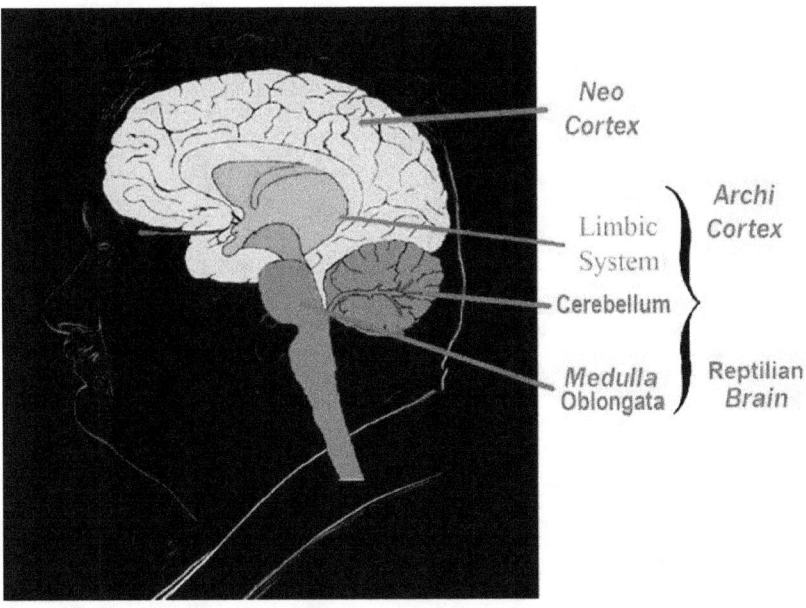

Neo Cortex

Archi Cortex

Limbic System

Cerebellum

Medulla Oblongata

Reptilian Brain

Figure 1 The Two Control Centers of the Brain: The Old and New.

The reptile vigorously defends its territory for food supply. One can, with equal vehemence, defend one's intellectual territory (diagnoses). The reptile also preens itself. The cosmetic, automotive, and fashion industries count on our preening. **(EGOSIM)**

The reptile shuns strangers and prefers to hang out with its own kind. We pick up clues from our colleagues and nurses about the merits of patients and unconsciously tune our diligence accordingly. **(LABELING)**

With sleep deprivation or with repeated threats to its territory or life, the reptile will eventually become apathetic. Our sleep center is in our reptilian brain. **(RESIGNATION, APATHY)**

The reptile behaves like a spoiled child. "Give me what I want and I want it now." **(CONVENIENCE)**

The reptile embraces certainty and abhors uncertainty. Uncertainty is inconvenient; certainty is convenient. (**CONVENIENCE**)

Figure 2 below outlines the progression toward the Theorem of Attribution, namely: Error is an expression of our reptilian brain.

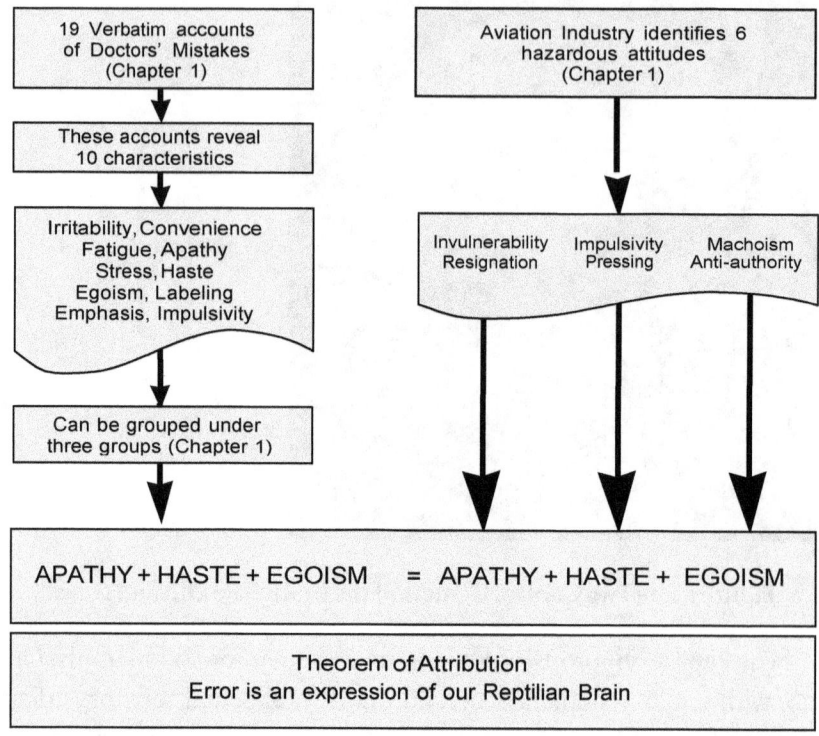

Figure 2 Outline of Theorem of Attribution of Error to the Reptilian Brain

When we mine the seam of our error, we are re-introduced to that mother lode of error, our reptilian brain, which has a surprisingly limited number of expressions. Is it possible to over-ride our reptilian brain? This question is explored in Chapter 2.

CHAPTER 2

Contending Against Reptilian Attachments

Is it possible to over-ride our reptilian brain? John Henry Cardinal Newman doubted it. "Quarry the granite rocks with razors, or moor the vessel with a thread of silk; then may you hope with such keen and delicate instruments as human knowledge and human reason to contend against those giants, the passions and pride of man." This is a bleak appraisal of the ability of our new brain to combat our non-reflecting lower brain. The existentialists, on the other hand, write of our freedom to respond. Sartre says that, "the one thing we can't avoid is choice." In his book, *"From Death Camp to Existentialism,"* Dr. Viktor Frankl, reflecting on his years as a prisoner in different Nazi death camps, showed how different prisoners responded to the same system.[20]

"The experiences of camp life show that man does have a choice of action. There were enough examples, often of a heroic nature, which proved that apathy could be overcome, irritability suppressed. Man can preserve a vestige of spiritual freedom, of independence of mind, even in such terrible conditions of psychic and physical stress.

We who lived in the concentration camps can remember the men who walked through the huts comforting others, giving away their last piece of bread. They may have been few in number, but they offer sufficient proof that everything can be taken away from man but one thing: the last of the human freedoms - to choose one's attitude in any given set of circumstances, to choose one's own way.

And there were always choices to make. Every day, every hour, offered the opportunity to make a decision which determined whether you would or would not submit to those powers which threatened to rob you of your very self, your inner freedom; which determined whether or not you would become the plaything of circumstance, renouncing freedom and dignity to become molded into the form of the typical inmate.

Even tough conditions such as lack of sleep, insufficient food and various mental stresses may suggest that the inmates were bound to react in certain ways. *In the final analysis it became clear that the sort of person the prisoner became was the result of an inner decision and not the result of camp influences alone.* Fundamentally, therefore, any man can even under such circumstances, decide what shall become of him - mentally and spiritually".[21] (italics mine).

Frankl claims that, though subjected to such profound depravity and despair, some could decide to respond with politeness not rudeness, with humor not dullness, with altruism not selfishness, in essence with the new brain not the reptilian one. Similarly, we have the choice, to respond with our new or old brain, to know or guess, to be attentive or inattentive. To improve our ability to respond with our new brain we have to first know and recognize the outward signs of the heightened reptilian attachment within. That is, when the reptile within first puckers its lips to show its fangs and hiss.

The Outward Signs of Heightened Reptilian Energy Within.

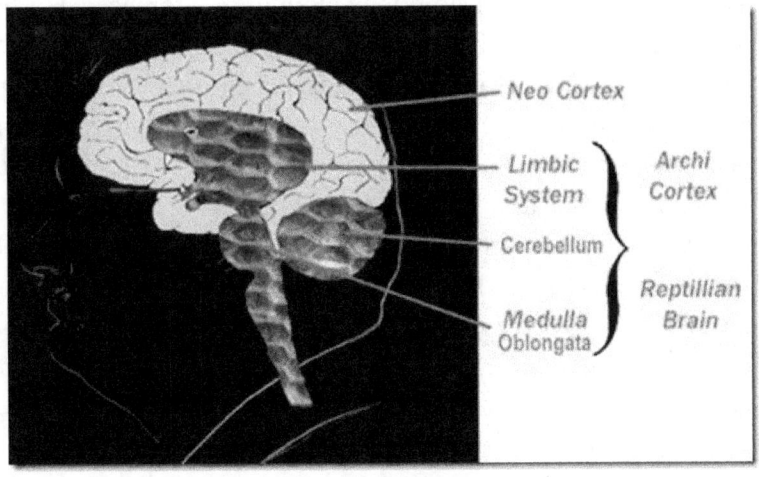

Figure 3 The Brain

The showing of fangs for the physician is expressed in the labeling (stigmatizing) of patients, be it with regard to their mores, plaintiveness, appearance, smell, status, story, frequency of presentation, manners or grammar. We also label patients by their triage placement and by pejorative labels bequeathed by staff, for example, the preview given by the nurse in the No. 7 account of the Ely Group (Chapter 1).

The hiss of the reptile within is one of impatience or irritability. John Keats, who trained as a physician, wrote of this impediment to quality work: "At once it struck me what quality went to form a Man of Achievement, especially in Literature and which Shakespeare possessed so enormously. I mean NEGATIVE CAPABILITY... that is, when a man is capable of being in uncertainties, mysteries, doubts, *without any irritable* reaching after fact and reason."[22] (Italics are mine). Both Keats's negative capability and Osler's imperturbability demand freedom from irritability.

Dr. Carey Chisholm's account "A Case Study in Error"[23] highlights both new brain and reptilian expressions in a clinical setting. It is instructive to read this richly-textured, thorough, and unusually fearless and frank account.

She is in a wheelchair, headed for room 15. Middle-aged, Caucasian, obese, and crying. Damp face cloth on her forehead. Husband is in tow, holding her handbag, looking detached. Chief complaint: "abdominal and leg pain by four days." Triage category 3. "Not sick "goes through my mind. We aren't very busy yet that morning, with quite a few residents and students just reporting for duty. Twenty minutes later, after five other new patients are picked up in front of her (the vaginal bleeding and cramps patient being preferentially rack-picked was the defining moment), my time threshold was exceeded and off I went to see her myself.

I walk into the room. The patient is in her pajamas, in her bathrobe with her slippers on. Why the hell can't the nurses ever get patients undressed?" goes through my mind. Mrs. X is wriggling and rolling from side to side on the bed, eyes closed, damp wash-cloth on her forehead, moaning frequently. "Not peritonitis" rolls through my head. "Not sick, at least not physically" slides up to the forebrain. "I'm DR. C, I understand that you have not been well for a few days," as I reach for the nurse's notes with the vital signs. Patient moans, and the husband steps to the plate. "Yeah, she'd been vomiting everything up for two days. It all started in her leg. Now her belly's been hurting just like the last time." Nurses notes: "fever, right leg pain, nausea and vomiting by two days." Vital signs: temperature 97°, pulse 100, respiratory rate 24, blood pressure 131/87, oxygen saturation 100% in room air. Meds: Effexor, Pepcid "Vital signs are normal, she's not too sick" crosses my mind.

I discount the leg pain, and head for the money (based on the husband's… "just like the last time"). "What's been wrong with her belly in the past?"

Her husband explains, while she continues to moan and roll from side to side. There is an umbilical hernia requiring repair in the upcoming months by a "plastic surgeon." She has had her appendix and gallbladder removed, and last winter had a tumor in her pelvis that they took out, along with all her female organs." "It wasn't cancer, though.

The wound got infected and she had had several operations. We fired her first two surgeons, and now she uses Dr. X X X at University Hos- pital. He's going to fix her hernia."

"Ah, bowel obstruction," I think. "How are you feeling right now?" Moans and crying with more rolling. I hold her shoulder. "Ma'am, I can't help you unless you talk to me. You look as though you're very uncomfortable. Tell me what symptoms you are having so I can help you to feel better." She starts to hyperventilate and moans faster. "What an excellent first patient for the day," I think. "Ma'am, are you having pain right now?" Then it comes, after about 30 seconds of silence and rapid breathing.... rolled on her side, in a semifetal position... a whiney whisper that raises the hair on my neck more effectively than fingernails on a chalkboard. "Yesssssss. Ohhhhhhhh. Ohhhhhhhhhh." "Ma'am, WHERE does it hurt?" (I know the answer even as I ask...). "Ohhhhhhhhhh. All over. Everywhere." The patient begins retching, and flicks her hands into the air, wrists wrangling. I give her an emesis basin. She spends about 2 minutes retching, but produces nothing. I wonder if this isn't simply for my benefit, or per- haps the husband's. Is she being abused? "Ma'am, I need to examine you to see what's wrong." As she continues to roll from side to side, I try to palpate her abdomen through her bathrobe and pajamas. I give the gurney a good rattle and shake her pelvis... no evident increase in pain ("no peritonitis" again rolls through my thoughts). Her belly doesn't feel distended and there is no involuntary guarding.

"I'm going to give you some medicine for the nausea and pain. I'm also going to give you some fluids through your vein and draw some blood studies. I need to look up your old records and see what they did earlier this year. I'll need you to get undressed and into a gown so that I can examine you." I order promethazine and diphenhy- dramine, deciding to wait on the opioid until after I sort out if it's nau- sea or pain that is causing such a fracas.

I look her up in our computerised database. Neither the name nor the medical record number comes up with any hits. I return to the room and verify that she was cared for here in the past. The husband thinks that her records are at University Hospital (these would be part

13

of our database). I wonder why she's not in the database.

Thirty minutes later it was discovered that her medical record number was entered incorrectly during registration and is corrected. The computer now provides more than 20 pages of records for me. I browse through these in between staffing two cases. "Fired" Drs. A and B, two of the nicest and most competent general surgeons on our medical staff, last February after her wound became infected. Admitted in May and July for presumed small bowel obstruction and underwent enterolysis. I go back to see her, 50 minutes after my initial encounter. Fetal position, moans are diminished. In a gown, still, with pajama bottoms and underwear on. I get more history… the nausea is now much better although the pain hasn't improved. It is periumbilical, colicky, radiates centrally to the umbilicus. Bowel movements by four times since yesterday without blood or diarrhoea, last six hours ago. No oral intake since noon yesterday due to nausea and emesis. Pain started in her right leg at the ankle and thigh and "migrated" into her abdomen. No peritoneal signs, no masses. She still resists efforts to examine her while she lies on her back. She says that this is "identical" to her episodes in May and July. I decide she must have an early bowel obstruction. Her leg is normal color and size, no effusion. Palpation doesn't seem to elicit pain. I decide to measure it. No tape measures in the room. I go to the next three adjacent rooms… no tape measures. I go to the nurses' station… they can't find one, but will hunt one down and put it in the room for me.

I remembered as I haven't ordered any labs since I wanted to first check her medical records and then got interrupted by a medical student as I was about to return to her room to place my orders. Now almost an hour into it, I order an acute abdominal series, complete blood count, basic metabolic profile, lipase, liver function tests, and urine. I wonder why the nurses didn't ask me if I wanted any labs when they started her intravenous. "Oh well, if I get her symptoms under control I may be able to put her in the observation unit and send her home later," I think.

I order morphine for her pain, and re-dose the promethazine shortly afterward when she complains to the nurse of worsening nausea. One hour later she vomits, so I order dolasetron (the nurses are now telling me that "she's high maintenance"). I know I won't be sending her home and note that the radiographs should be back along with her labs. No obstruction, mild elevation, and atelectasis right lung field (unchanged from the May and July chest radiographs that I look at), positive ketones in her urinary analysis, white cell count 11.000, hemoglobin and hematocrit fine, bicarbonate 15 with anion gap of 15. Lipase and liver function tests are normal except small elevation of alkaline phosphatase.

I enter the room to deliver news (three hours, 30 minutes after she arrived) and two more doses of morphine and one litre of normal saline later. She's back to rocking slowly back and forth, tearful, and has the whine going. "I'm sooooooooo siiiiiiiiiiick! Ohhhhhhhhhh." There are now an additional mother, aunt and sister along with the husband. No one looks too happy. I re-examine her abdomen…no change. I explain that I'll call her doctor and admit her to the hospital for a presumptive early small bowel obstruction.

Dr. X. X. X. is scrubbed in the operating room at University Hospital. I relay information to a doctor I do not know, second hand through a nurse whom I don't know. Dr. X. X. X. points out that he's a plastic surgeon and this isn't in his expertise area. I ask him whom I should contact instead, because she fired general surgeons here. He doesn't know with "this new system" and all. Ball back in my court…..

I return to the room and explain that we'll have to go doctor shopping, after some discussion, they agree to go with the on-call surgeon. (I hope that it isn't Dr. A or B!). The mother stops me as I go to leave the room. "Aren't you going to do something about her leg?" I quickly re-examine it….soft, good color and temperature, doesn't feel firm. I remembered that I haven't measured it, and also that there still is no tape measure in her room. It appears identical to the other leg. Palpation now seems to be subjectively uncomfortable anywhere that I touch it. I explain that I am uncertain what is causing her leg pain, but that I'm focusing on her abdominal pain. Mom says, "Her father died from a blood clot in his leg." I order a venous duplex ultrasound. I look at her flow sheet…no repeat vital signs. I ask the nurses to repeat her vital signs. This is done four hours and 30 minutes after her initial

15

set. Still afebrile pulse 79, BP 139/82, respiratory rate 22. The following thoughts go through my mind: "At least it appears that it's nothing big I'm missing....she has pain out of proportion to her examination, and says it's identical to two prior episodes. I can't have been missing dead gut. Let's get this ultrasound (mainly for Mom's benefit), get a surgeon, and get her and her family out of here before the nurses hang me."

One hour later, she returns from ultrasound. She's rolling again, and the moans seem to be at a new fingernail-stretching tone (I think, "for the benefit of her family"). She says her abdominal pain is even worse. Her examination (in between rolls) is unchanged. I decide to unequivocally rule out dead gut and order a venous lactate, an abdominal computer tomography (CT) with contrast, and more morphine. I admit her to one of the partners of the fired surgeons. He sends his physician's assistant to see her. History and physical and orders are written by the physician's assistant. I begin to relax she's now somebody else's problem patient.

Ultrasound calls: Deep venous thrombosis throughout the entire femoral system. I check for anticoagulant risks, explain to the family that we know the reason for the leg pain, and order enoxaparin. They all seem to have an "I told you so" look about them (or is that simply my imagination?). I wonder how the day would have gone if I had rack-picked the vaginal bleeder instead of this lady as my first patient. "Could a medical student have screwed this up as badly as I did?"

A hospitalist is requested after I call the surgeon and point out the new issue of the deep vein thrombosis. He quickly sees the patient. This delays the patient's oral contrast administration, which ultimately necessitates a nasogastric tube placement. He mentions to me that she's "difficult." As he walks over to write his note, he says, "Pretty wild that she drove all the way from Florida[24] seven days ago with only two stops..." ("Gee, that would have been a nice piece of history to elicit," I think. "What an embarrassment.")

My shift is over. I turn her over to my partner as pending abdominal CT and venous lactate...."if there's dead gut, her surgeons need to be called." Otherwise, orders are written, including pain medication and anti-emetics.

I wake up at two o'clock in the morning in a sweat. 'Dead gut. I missed dead gut.' Or maybe worse, necrotizing fasciitis." And I gave her enoxaparin…the surgeon will love that when he goes to the operating room." I toss and turn for another two hours before going back to sleep. I decide that sharing of this would be of interest for some and cathartic for me.

Discharge diagnosis: Ileus, inflammatory bowel, right lower extremity deep vein thrombosis, multiple pulmonary emboli bilaterally, ventral hernia.

This ends Dr. Chisholm's account.

Reflections upon Dr. Chisholm's account: [25]

Both Dr. Chisholm and I awoke with grave concerns about our respective patients' well-being, an unease we did not fully appreciate when we were tending our patients. During sleep we are free of fatigue, of inconvenience, of labels, of haste, and of our self-esteem. Our resting reptilian brain frees up space for the new brain to rotate through possibilities.[26] In sleep, we escape that tyrant, the reptilian brain, and we reach imperturbability, the quality which Osler prized.

Dr. Chisholm and I, and the nurses tending our patients, were inattentive to the abnormal vital signs of our patients. The skill of attention is neglected in schools and in higher institutions of learning. Acquiring the skill of attention will be addressed in Chapter 4 (Third Skill of the NewMind Response™: maintaining vigilance to the task at hand).

The dislike Dr. Chisholm experienced toward his patient is stiffened by his uncertainties about his examination. (I have found that my dislike toward my patient was more a reflection of my doubts than the patient's personality). It is probable that the hospitalist did not dislike the same patient because the diagnosis was established.

It is a lesson for the learning that it was not Dr. Chisholm's knowledge but his character that steered him on the correct path. The signs of reptilian expressions and new brain activities in Dr. Chisholm's ac-

17

count are worth considering.

Reptilian Expressions in Dr. Chisholm's Account

Labeling:
The nurse labeled the patient: "she was high maintenance." "Eyes rolling" implies that the patient was judged to be over-reacting. Dr. Chisholm noted that her husband "looked detached". One could sense that Dr. Chisholm felt that his patient was being dramatic. In reading the account, I felt that his patient was dramatic. Labels, like diagnoses, are easier to apply than remove.

Irritability:
Dr. Chisholm appears to be irritated by:
the rack-pickers
the dressed patient
the missing tape measure
the nurses' irritability

Egoism:
Only once is Dr. Chisholm concerned about the nurses' opinion of him: "get her and her family out of here before the nurses hang me."

Haste:
From the beginning of Dr. Chisholm's shift to the admission of his patient, time prods him.

We learn that 20 minutes of stalling catapults him into action.

The tape measure hunt and the dressed patient delay him. These delays irritate him, yet he could wait 20 minutes before seeing any patient.

"I discount the leg pain, and head for the money...." Dr. Chisholm is irritated by the delay in getting a receiving physician for his patient. "Now it is almost an hour before I order...."

Again we learn "I enter the room to deliver news (3 hours, 30 minutes after she arrived)."

The New Brain Initiatives of Dr. Chisholm

Humility:
The opposite to egoism is humility. Dr. Chisholm had the humility both to face the nurses' critique of his "security blanket" orders, and to accept guidance from the patient's mother. By contrast, I refused guidance from my patient's relatives and nurse. Pilots say, "It's not who's right but what's right."

Doing the Inconvenient:
In the learning points listed at the end of this article, Dr. Chisholm reflects: "Finally, **my policy of repeated trips to the bedside of the patients whom I don't like** eventually saved me in this case." (Bold type mine). Dr. Chisholm returned four times to his patient. Four returns to one's failure requires both gumption and humility, both new brain initiatives. As Nikos Kazantzakis prays in his autobiography: "May I always return to where I have failed."[27]

In Zen and the Art of Motorcycle Maintenance, Robert Pirsig writes about gumption.

"If you are going to repair a motorcycle, an adequate supply of gumption is the first and most important tool. If you haven't got that you might as well gather up your tools and put them away, because they won't do you any good... Gumption is the psychic gasoline that keeps the whole thing going. If you haven't got it there's no way the motorcycle can possibly be fixed. But if you have it and know how to keep it, there's absolutely no way in this world that that motorcycle can keep from getting fixed. It's bound to happen. Therefore the thing that must be monitored at all times and preserved before anything, is gumption."[28]

Dr. Chisholm had the gumption to persist through his doubt and failure.

Conclusion:

It is reassuring that Dr. Chisholm, by his gumption to do the inconvenient, by his doubting and by his humility to accept the mother's challenge, was able to diagnose this patient despite the fervent reptilian expressions he experienced. This action supports Frankl's claim that we have a choice, a choice to counter those giants, the passions and pride of man.

Table 1 below shows a more detailed list of the activities and characteristics of the reptilian brain and the new brain.

Activities and Characteristics of the Reptilian Brain	Activities and Characteristics of the New Brain
Labeling, liking and disliking others and processes. Critical of others.	Non-judgmental of others. Critical of oneself, self-questioning.
Haste, pressing, impulsivity, fretting about time.	Content about the present activity. Not focused on time.
Favoring the convenient.	Having the resolve to do the inconvenient.
Apathetic, complacent, taking short-cuts, ambushing the symptoms which are the least strenuous for us.	Treating this patient like one would wish to be treated.
Distracted, inattentive to the task at hand.	Vigilant to the task at hand.
Promptly dismiss doubt. Make assumptions, lounge, guess.	Give doubt an honest hearing (See Ch. 12).
Egoism, one's self-esteem can interfere with decisions taken.	To advocate the patient's interests, not one's own self-esteem. To have the humility to take it on the chin for the patient.
Irritability.	Imperturbability. Negative Capability.
Hearing, not listening. Interrupts frequently, talks over.	Active Listening (See Ch. 11).

Reacting.	Self-reflection and self-monitoring.
Naming as in diagnosing. Emphatic Expressions.	Undoing, un-naming, retracing. Tentative, open to other ideas.
No professional courtesy.	Professional courtesy and understanding.

Table 1 Activities and Characteristics of the Reptilian and the New Brains

By reducing attachment to the reptilian brain, the physician's new brain is unfurled, enabling it to take in challenging data regarding the patient's presentation, becoming more objective. This reduction of the reptilian brain's attachments and the consequent enhancement of the new brain attachment, I call the NewMind Response™. The Theorem of Attachments and the NewMind Response™ are outlined in Figure 4 below.

> **FIRST ASSUMPTION**
> The total energy of both the Reptilian Brain and the New Brain is constant
> (For exception see Chapter 3)

> **SECOND ASSUMPTION**
> Likewise, the total of one's attachment to the
> Reptilian Brain and the New Brain is also constant Kta
> Kta= A.R.B. + A.N.B.

> **The Theorem of Attachments**
> The more attachments we have to one brain
> the fewer we have to the other
> (For exceptions see Chapter 3)

> **NewMind Response™**
> To reduce error we need to reduce attachment to
> our Reptilian Brain, thereby increasing space for our
> New Brain activity.

Figure 4 Outline to Theorem of Attachments and the NewMind Reponse™

The next chapter outlines how to strive for the NewMind Response™

CHAPTER 4

Striving toward The NewMind Response™

*We are what we repeatedly do. Excellence, then, is not an act,
but a habit. -Aristotle*

To reduce attachment to the reptilian brain and enhance attach
ment to the new brain demands the honing of **three skills:**
SKILL 1: the self-monitoring of one's attachment to the reptilian
brain (**4 steps**)
SKILL 2: the curbing of one's attachment to the reptilian brain
(**2 steps**) and
SKILL 3: vigilance to the task at hand.

These three skills are difficult to master because we are attempting
with a new brain (designed only a few million years ago) to overcome
an old brain, entrenched for 200 million years. This old brain has pre-
eminence and is hardwired to assumptions and snap reactions.[32] Therefore the NewMind Response™ is not automatic, but with practice is
attainable.

**SKILL 1: Self-monitoring one's attachment to the reptil-
ian brain by building and using one's Irritability
Barometer.**

To self-monitor attachment to the reptilian brain, one can measure one's irritability level. How? We need to create an **irritability barometer** which can score our responses to common irritants at home, commuting, and at work. Building, calibrating and using one's irritability barometer takes four steps:
- Make a list of frequent irritants
- Categorize one's different levels of responses to irritants
- Match one's usual responses to the frequent irritants listed in step one
- Practice monitoring levels of responses to common irritants

Step 1: Make a list of frequent irritants
Make a list of the frequent irritants at home, commuting, and at work. The more irritants we identify, the more often we can employ our irritability barometer.

A list might look like this:

At Home:
Loud music at home or next door
Children bickering
Toys in the driveway
Clothes lying on the floor
Complaints about the inconsequential
Failure to relay messages
Failure to do chores
Doing chores
Computer malfunctioning
Telemarketing calls
Barking dogs
Shortage of food supplies
Wasting food
Wasting electricity
Balking at homework or bedtime
Door slamming

Taking long showers
Bills to be paid

Commuting:
Delays by partner or children to leave the house
Car refuses to start
Ice and snow on the windshields
The snow plough has just blocked the end of the driveway
Detours to work
Red traffic lights
Lane-hoppers
Slow drivers
Difficulty finding parking
Fuel low in tank.

At Work:
Being put on hold on the telephone
Delay in getting results, instruments
Delay in starting surgery or office
Colleague "cherry-picking" the charts
Boisterous behavior at work
Annoying, lazy staff
Complaints about the inconsequential
Interruptions
Discourteous, importuning or truculent patients
Dressed patients
Illegible handwriting
Reflex hammer, tape measure, etc. not at hand.

Step 2: Categorize one's different levels of responses to irritants.

We can classify our responses to common irritants into four categories, from neutral to severe. A classification might look like this:

Neutral response: Respond with humor or view the irritant from three months into the future, like Viktor Frankl described. (See Chapter 9)

Mild irritability: Begin to blame, criticize or dislike/ anyone or anything, or to sigh, roll the eyes, and become sarcastic.

Moderate irritability: To look at the time, to quicken one's pace, to interrupt, to be preoccupied with formulating a response; to change one's voice pitch or tone, to tighten one's jaw or paw; to lean forward in one's chair, and movements to become twitchy.

Severe irritability: One's voice becomes edgy-growling, one's breath quickens, one doesn't listen, one talks over the other person. Regardless of what is said, one takes the opposite point of view. One squirms, sweats, changes stance, has the urge to stand up and show the patient the door.

Step 3: Match one's usual responses to the frequent irritants listed in step one.

Strive to establish an accurate base line of one's **usual** responses to each of the irritants. As with most instruments, the more one calibrates one's irritability barometer, the more accurate it becomes. See Table 2 for examples.

	Humor	Mild	Moderate	Severe
Loud music at home or next door				
Children bickering				
Clothes lying on the floor				
Failure to relay messages				
Failure to do chores				
Doing chores oneself				
Computer malfunctioning				
Telemarketing calls				
Shortage of food supplies				
Door slamming				
Wasting electricity				
Balking at homework / bedtime				
Taking long showers				
Not turning lights off				
Outstanding bills				
Toys in the driveway				
Complaints about the inconsequential.				

Table 2 Reader's Usual Responses to Irritants

	Humor	Mild	Moderate	Severe
Delays leaving the house				
Ice on the windshield				
Bus or metro delays				
Red traffic lights				
Lane-hoppers				
Difficulty finding parking				

List of Irritants At Home
Check your usual Responses
Irritants Commuting

	Humor	Mild	Moderate	Severe
Delay in getting results				
Colleague cherry-picking the charts				
Boisterous behavior at work				
Annoying, lazy staff				
Interruptions to help colleague or to socialize				

Check your usual Responses

	Humor	Mild	Moderate	Severe
Discourteous, demanding or truculent patients				
Delay in turn-over time				
Complaints about the inconsequential				
Wait for proper instruments				
Pen stolen or misplaced				
Being put on hold on the telephone				

Irritants at Work
Check your usual Responses

Step 4: Practice monitoring levels of responses to common irritants.

Place the list of irritants with their corresponding standard levels of response: in a desk at home, in the glove compartment of the car, and in your notebook at work. Practice acknowledging each irritant as it occurs and noting the level of response it elicits.

Practice noting one's irritants with their levels of responses. If the response to a standard irritant is **more than usual,** then reptilian influence is stronger, mischief is afoot. This step is crucial to glimpse the chameleon-like heightened reptilian response within. To identify and counter the source or sources of heightened reptilian response within, proceed to Skill 2 below.

But firstly, here's an example of my monitoring attachment to the reptilian brain. I used to be upset by a staff member of the emergency department. He would sit at the center of the charting desk of the nursing station and would talk constantly to anyone around about his dog and cat, his motor bike and car, his friends and the weather, his snow-blower and the potholes in the street, his lawn-mower and the news, his family and the real estate prices, his sagging belly, and even his clothesline. I had silently nick-named him "The Radio". At first "The Radio" would upset me, but then I realized that he was a standardized irritant and that I could use him to score my irritability response at any moment that he was there. Should my response to "The Radio" increase, then my reptilian brain was more energetic. The cause for this heightened response could then be traced through Step one of Skill 2 below.

SKILL 2. Curbing the heightened attachment to the Reptilian Brain (Two Steps)

Step 1: Identify the source(s) of the heightened reptilian attachment.

(Irritability acts as a vital sign. Vital signs when abnormal tell us that something is amiss, it does not say what is amiss).

There are four sources for heightened attachment to the reptilian brain. These are: Haste, Egoism, Apathy (from either burnout or sleep deprivation), and Doubt. Which of these attitudes is present? Just ask:

Am I rushing?

Am I tired?

Am I concerned about my self-image?

Am I doubting? (Doubting, a new brain activity, is an irritant to the reptilian brain which craves certainty).

Once one has identified the source, counter it unless the source is due to doubt.

Step 2: Countering the source of the heightened reptilian attachment.

The Crew Resource Management Manual for pilots recommends positive Responses for the Hazardous Attitudes.[33] They call these responses "antidotes". By repeating to oneself these antidotes one can counter the reptilian attitude. Note that doubting does not require an antidote, because it is a new brain activity. See Table 3 for specific antidotes. For generic antidotes see Chapter 13.

Haste	"Not so fast. Think first."
Egoism	It's not who is right, but what's right. The patient's well-being is more important than my self-esteem.
Tired, apathetic, "What's the use?"	"I am not helpless, I can make a difference."
Labeling	Will impede more than help in diagnosing the patient.
Convenience	Effort is the clarity we seek.[34] The correct action is often inconvenient. Stellar action is always inconvenient.[35]

Table 3 Specific Antidotes

Reptilian Attitudes   **Specific Antidotes**

Doubt is an inconvenience, but should be acknowledged, welcomed and explored. The response to doubt is revising the history and physical examination, opening the differential diagnoses and considering compounding factors. Doubting also can signal one's limitations or incompetence and the need to consult a specialist. (Again, Chapter 12 is devoted to doubting).

SKILL 3: Maintaining vigilance to the task at hand

Maintaining attention is also a skill, like hitting a tennis ball or playing the guitar. The more one practices, the more adept one becomes. Regrettably, many of us have seldom practiced being attentive. It is neglected in schools, colleges and universities. We practice inattention not attention: the jogger with the iPod, the driver with the cell phone or the radio on, the reader with the music or the TV on.[36] Attention is an under-exercised muscle. We can pump this muscle throughout the day by concentrating solely on what we are now doing.

Being vigilant to the task at hand: In the morning

As we get out of bed, think of easing ourselves up and lifting off the bed-clothes. And when we shower, strive to think only of the shower and washing oneself. And when we dress, think of the movements in- volved. And when we prepare breakfast, think of pouring the cereal into the bowl, of pouring the milk, of getting the spoon, of folding the paper of the cereal container, of sitting. Think of lifting the spoon to the cereal and bringing it to the mouth.

Being vigilant to the task at hand: Driving to work

When leaving the house, strive to be aware of closing the door, and of locking it. When walking to the car, think of the steps one is taking. When opening the door think of pressing the handle and opening the door. Be vigilant to sitting into the seat and to buckling up, and the same for starting the engine. When driving to work, just concentrate on the traffic and responses to irritants. Practice attention only to your driving. Such attention is twice blessed: it helps to avert an accident and is also practice for vigilance to the task at hand.

Being vigilant to the task at hand: At work

Upon picking up a chart, read the nurse's comments, and the vital signs. Ask one's self, are these vital signs normal? When listening to a patient, sit down, where appropriate, and listen. The art of listening will be addressed in Chapter 11.When inspecting, auscultating, and palpating organs, practice vigilance to the task at hand, like the focus of Osler in Figure 5.

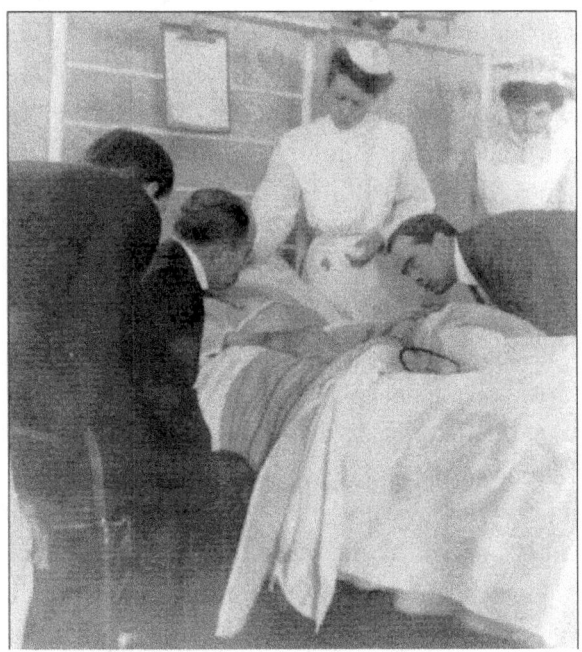

Figure 5 Osler observing the Patient.

Being vigilant to the task at hand: In the evening

At home, when washing a dish or a bowl, think only of washing the dish or the bowl. One might find oneself planning what to do when finished the chore. The exercise, however, is to focus on each of the tasks of washing up, as they are encountered until they are finished. Be there, be present, with the bowl and the cleaning of the bowl. When the radio is on just sit down and listen to the radio, do nothing else.

Conclusion:

At first, strive to be attentive to the task at hand, realize that attention is difficult to maintain, distractions abound, uninvited random thoughts appear, linger and are replaced by others, like the TV monitor at the mercy of a teenager with the remote control. But practice improves one's focus on the task at hand.

As mentioned earlier, inattention is transient blindness and transient deafness. Inattention or daydreaming is easy. Attention, on the other hand, demands one's will and full concentration.

These callisthenics tune one's attention muscles for vigilance to the task at hand at work. (Just as callisthenics promotes physical vigour and grace, likewise appropriate mental callisthenics promotes mental vigour and grace).

The more one practices them, the easier it becomes to be attentive to the task at hand. At first, it was difficult to remember to fasten the seat belts in the car, but with practice it became a habit, and now when the seat belt is unbuckled, one feels ill-at-ease until buckled up. Similarly, the more one practices attention to the task at hand, the more one notices its absence. When one has difficulty being vigilant to the task at hand, the more likely one has heightened attachment to the reptilian brain. Curbing one's attachment to the reptilian brain and being vigilant to the task at hand are mutually enhancing.

Summary: The patient deserves that the physician be both patient and vigilant to the task at hand. A medical aphorism instructs: have the eye of an eagle, the ear of a dog, the heart of a lion and the hand of a mother. To achieve these ideals, many need to practice vigilance to the task at hand, self-monitoring the irritability barometer, discovering the source of heightened irritability, and dosing with the appropriate antidote or antidotes.

CHAPTER 5

An Example of the NewMind Response™ from Dr. A. J. Cronin

*"The real cycle you're working on is a cycle called yourself.....
working on a motorcycle is to become part of a process, to
achieve an inner peace of mind." from the epigraph to Robert
M. Pirsig's Zen and the Art of Motorcycle Maintenance.*

The example, set in a small Welsh mining town, is from
"The Citadel" by A. J. Cronin.

"On the following Friday, at six o'clock in the morning, Dr. Andrew
Manson was awakened by a knocking on his bedroom door. It was Annie, and
very red about the eyes, offering him a note.

Andrew tore open the envelope. It was a message from Doctor Bramwell:

"Come round at once. I want you to help certify a dangerous lunatic." Annie
struggled with her tears.

"It's Emrys, Doctor. A dreadful thing has happened. I do hope you'll come
down quick, like."

Andrew threw on his things in three minutes. Accompanying him down the
road, Annie told him as best she could about Emrys. He had been ill and un- like
himself for three weeks, but during the night he had turned violent, and gone
clean out of his mind. He had set upon his wife with a bread-knife. Olwen (Emrys'
wife) had just managed to escape by running into the street in her night- gown. The
sensational story was sufficiently distressing as Annie brokenly related it,
hurrying beside him in the grey light of morning, and there seemed little he

could add, by way of consolation, to alter it. They reached the Hughes's house. In the front room Andrew found Doctor Bramwell, unshaven, without his collar and tie, wearing a serious air, seated at the table, pen in hand. Before him was a bluish paper form, half filled in.

"Ah, Manson! Good of you to come so quickly. A bad business this. But it won't keep you long."

"What's up?"

"Hughes has gone mad. I think I mentioned to you a week ago I was afraid of it. Well! I was right. Acute mania." Bramwell rolled the words over his tongue with tragic grandeur. "Acute homicidal mania. We'll have to get him into Pontynewdd straight away. That means two signatures on the certificate, mine and yours - the relatives wanted me to call you in. You know the procedure, don't you?"

"Yes." Andrew nodded. "What's your evidence?"

Bramwell began, clearing his throat, to read what he had written upon the form. It was a full, flowing account of certain of Hughes's actions during the previous week, all of them conclusive of mental derangement. At the end of it Bramwell raised his head. "Clear evidence, I think!"

"It sounds pretty bad," Andrew answered slowly. "Well! I'll take a look at him."

"Thanks, Manson. You'll find me here when you're finished," And he began to add further particulars to the form.

Emrys Hughes was in bed, and seated beside him - in case restraint should be necessary - were two of his mates from the mine.

Standing by the foot of the bed was Olwen, her pale face, ordinarily so pert and lively, now ravaged by weeping. Her attitude was so overwrought, the atmosphere of the room so dim and tense, that Andrew had a momentary thrill of coldness, almost of fear.

He went over to Emrys, and at first he hardly recognized him. The change was not gross; it was Emrys true enough, but a blurred and altered Emrys, his features coarsened in some subtle way. His face seemed swollen, the nostrils thickened, the skin waxy, except a faint reddish patch that spread across the nose. His whole appearance was heavy, apathetic. Andrew spoke to him. He muttered a reply. Then, clenching his hands, he came out with a tirade of aggressive nonsense, which, added to Bramwell's account, made the case for his removal only too conclusive.

A silence followed. Andrew felt that he ought to be convinced. Yet, inexplicably, he was not satisfied. Why, why, he kept asking why should Hughes talk like this? Supposing the man had gone out of his mind, what was the cause of it all? He had always been a happy, contented man - no worries, easygoing, amicable. Why, without apparent reason, had he changed to this?

There must be a reason, Manson thought doggedly; symptoms just don't happen of themselves. Staring at the swollen features before puzzling for some solution of the conundrum, he instinctively reached out and touched the swollen face, noting subconsciously, as he did so, that the pressure of his finger left no dent on his cheek.

All at once, electrically, a terminal vibrated in his brain. Why didn't the swelling pit on pressure? Because - now it was his heart that jumped! - because it was not true oedema, but myxoedema. He had it! No, no, he must not rush. Firmly, he caught hold of himself. He must not be a plunger, wildly leaping to conclusions. He must go cautiously, slowly, be sure!

Curbing himself, he lifted Emrys' hand. Yes, the skin was dry and rough, the fingers slightly thickened at the ends. Temperature – it was subnormal. Methodically he finished the examination, fighting back each successive wave of elation. Every sign and every symptom - they fitted as superbly as a complex jig- saw puzzle. The clumsy speech, dry skin, spatulate fingers, the swollen inelastic face, the defective memory, slow mentation, the attacks of irritability culminating in an outburst of homicidal violence. Oh! The triumph of the completed picture was sublime.

Rising, he went down to the parlour, where Doctor Bramwell, standing on the hearthrug with his back to the fire, greeted him: -

"Well? Satisfied? The pen's on the table."

"Look here, Bramwell - " Andrew kept his eyes averted, battling to keep impetuous triumph from his voice. "I don't think we ought to certify Hughes."

"Eh, what?" Gradually the blankness left Bramwell's face. He exclaimed in hurt astonishment: "But the man's out of his mind!"

"That's not my view," Andrew answered in a level tone, still stopping down his excitement, his elation. It was not enough that he had diagnosed the case. He must handle Bramwell gently, try not to antagonize him. "In my opinion Hughes is only sick in mind because he's sick in body. I feel that he's suffering from thyroid deficiency - an absolutely straight case of myxoedema."

Bramwell stared at Andrew glassily. Now, indeed, he was dumbfounded. He made several efforts to speak - a queer sound, like snow falling off a roof.

"After all," Andrew went on persuasively, his eyes on the hearth-rug, "Pon-

37

tynewdd is such a sink of a place. Once Hughes gets in there he'll never get out. And if he does he'll carry the stigma of it all his life. Suppose we try pushing thyroid into him first?"

"Why, Doctor," Bramwell quavered, "I don't see - "

"Think of the credit for you," Andrew cut in quickly. "If you should get him well again. Don't you think it's worth it? Come on now, I'll call in Mrs. Hughes. She's crying her eyes out because she thinks Emrys is going away. You can explain we're going to try a new treatment."

Before Bramwell could protest Andrew went out of the room. A few minutes later, he came back with Mrs. Hughes. Planted on the hearthrug he informed Olwen in his best manner "that there might still be a ray of hope" while, behind his back, Andrew made a neat tight ball of the certificate and threw it in the fire. Then he went out to telephone to Cardiff for thyroid.

There was a period of quivering anxiety, several days of agonized suspense, before Hughes began to respond to the treatment. But once it started, that response was magical. Emrys was out of bed in a fortnight, and back at his work at the end of two months. He came round one evening to the surgery at Bryngower, lean and active, accompanied by the smiling Olwen, to tell Andrew he had never felt better in his life.

Reflections on Cronin's case of hypothyroidism

Reptilian activity

Haste and signs of irritability are almost absent from Manson's account, contrasting with both Dr. Chisholm's and my accounts. Where we find reptilian brain expression, we also find that Dr. Manson recognizes its presence and uses an effective antidote, for example, Manson's rush to name.

"He had it! No, no, he must not rush. Firmly, he caught hold of himself. He must not be a plunger, wildly leaping to conclusions. He must go cautiously, slowly, be sure! Curbing himself..."

And,

"Methodically he finished the examination, fighting back each successive wave of elation."

New Brain Activity

To doubt

The patient is framed and diagnosed by Dr. Bramwell as "Acute Homicidal Mania" and the symptoms of psychosis seemed a "no-brainer" for committal to a psychiatric hospital, yet Manson questioned what caused the change in his patient? Manson is able to acknowledge his own doubting and give it free rein. Cronin introduced Manson's doubting as silence:

"A silence followed. Andrew felt that he ought to be convinced. Yet, inexplicably, he was not satisfied. Why, why, he kept asking why should Hughes talk like this? Supposing the man had gone out of his mind, what was the cause of it all? He had always been a happy, contented man no worries, easygoing, amicable. Why, without apparent reason, had he changed to this?"

Has the gumption to do the inconvenient

"Manson thought doggedly, symptoms just don't happen by themselves."
"Methodically he finished the examination, ..."

Vigilance to the Task at Hand

When Manson looks at Emyrs' face, he is able to both appreciate it and then have the space to reflect upon it and Emyrs' demeanor. *"His face seemed swollen, the nostrils thickened, the skin waxy, except a faint reddish patch that spread across the nose. His whole appearance was heavy, apathetic."* Not only does he inspect the skin, but he also notes that it does not pit. (The hand of a mother). He is vigilant to the task at hand. If I had examined the skin of my patient with the volvulus, I might have noted that it tented[37] from dehydration.

Contrasting Doctors?

Both Bramwell and Manson practiced under the same system[38] and arrived at different diagnoses about the same patient. Bramwell was encrusted with reputation, experience, and knowledge while Manson was a recent medical graduate. Reputation, knowledge and experience, however, were trumped by doubting, vigilance to the task at hand, and self-monitoring and curbing reptilian activity and doing the inconvenient.

What drove Manson to be diligent and self-reflective? Cronin answers in the introduction to this parable: *"Manson was young enough to create in fancy a constant situation wherein she (Christine, a woman he admired) observed him at his cases, watched his careful methods, his scrupulous examinations, commended him for the searching accuracy of his diagnosis. Any temptation to scamp a visit, to reach a conclusion without first sounding the patient's chest, was met by the instant thought: "Lord, no! What would she think of me if I did that?...*

"He (Manson) admitted to himself that he still knew practically nothing. Yet he was teaching himself to think for himself, to look behind the obvious in an effort to find the proximate cause. Never before had he felt himself so powerfully attracted to the scientific ideal. He prayed that he might never become slovenly or mercenary, never to jump to conclusions, never to write "the mixture as before." He wanted to find out, to be scientific, to be worthy of Christine."

What is your motive? Though it is easy for the pilot to be motivated for excellence, doctors have to create their own motives for excellence, remembering that excellence is always inconvenient.

In fairness, Manson saw the miner for the first time in the full bloom of the disease; he had the advantage over Bramwell. It is easier to diagnose a disease in its maturity than in its infancy. A Chinese saying expresses this: "happy is the physician who sees the tail and not the head of the disease." The patient, however, is happier when the physician recognizes the beginning of the disease.

There's the story of one doctor asking another at a medical conference, "when did your wife begin treatment for her hyperthyroidism?" The questioned doctor looked with prompted eyes to recognize the bulging eyes of his wife. Signs and symptoms can stalk and overtake us. They had stalked Bramwell.

Is not our work like that of the detective? We gather data and then afterward look at the suspects in turn. (Let the ears and the eyes do the work before grey matter). Attention to details is necessary for both the

40

diagnostician and detective. How do we know when our detecting fever is cold or hot? How can we tell? Only the individual can, by standing outside oneself and self-monitoring like Manson had.

We are all blessed with the same organs to see, hear and touch. At- tention is required for these organs to look, listen and palpate. The art his- torian, James Elkins expresses the paradox, "blindness is not the opposite of vision, it is its constant companion."[39] And by extension, deafness is not the opposite of listening, it is its constant companion; and numbness is not the opposite of palpating, it is also its constant companion.

An example of blindness co-existing with vision follows. A colleague brought an X-ray to a consultant radiologist for his opinion. The X-ray was a lateral view of the cervical spine of a patient who endured trauma. The radiologist could not find anything wrong and pro- ceeded to point out all the intact alignments of the vertebral structures. My colleague then asked, "where is his head?" The injured man had been decapitated. Blindness is a constant companion of vision. Another physician when focusing on the neck of the femur missed the adjoining fracture of a pubic ramus.

I was one of about forty physicians attending a radiology teaching session in Vancouver. The radiologist showed a series of chest X-rays and invited diagnoses. He cycled through mediastinal and pulmonary cases. After several chest X-rays, we could not find the pathology on one. Finally after two to three minutes, the presenter showed us the transverse of a humerus. Blindness is a constant companion of vision. Bramwell had coupled symptom to diagnosis like vowels in a diphthong.[40] I had resolved to give symptoms more space to grow, unburdened with a diagnosis. Yet I continued to couple symptom to diagnosis: otitis media when I read earache; pharyngitis for sore throat. In short, I was addicted to coupling symptoms to diagnosis. How can one, in the fire of our agendas, learn to find the dieresis to pry symp- tom from diagnosis? Creating this separation, this space, will be dis- cussed: in "A Taoist Space for Diagnosing" (Chapter 10), Listening to the Whisper of Doubt Within (Chapter 12) and "A Physician Prepares to Meet the Patient" (Chapter 14).

PART II: BARRIERS TO GOOD WORK
Introduction to Barriers to Good Work

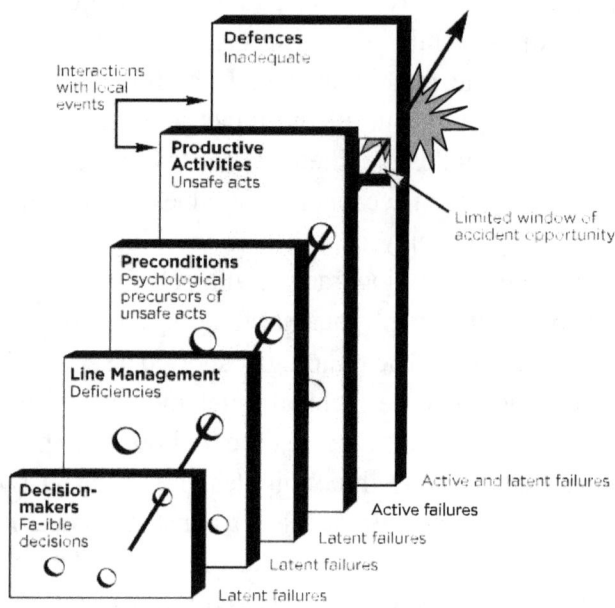

Figure 6 The Swiss Cheese Model

Relating the Swiss Cheese Model to Medical Performance

James Reason, at the The Second Halifax Symposium on Health-care Safety, discussed the barriers to error that exist in complex systems like nuclear plants and the aviation industry.[41] He portrayed these barriers as walls, walls lined up in a row, standing independently against error. These walls, however, have holes in them that allow error to penetrate. Should these holes line up then error can proceed uninterrupted and a mishap or accident can occur. He called the model, "The Swiss Cheese Model", Figure 6.

Regrettably this model does not transpose to the medical setting because there are few barriers to error in medicine. Unlike pilots, most doctors are unencumbered by regulations. For example:

- A doctor sees 173 patients in a twenty-four hour shift at a hospital.
- Some doctors book patients every five minutes.[42]
- Another has taken call for six months without a break.
- Some nurses work 12 hour shifts through the night from 7 PM to 7AM.
- Surgeons, intensivists, internists and anesthetists, when on call, can be expected to work for 24 hours, sometimes with little or no rest.
- Some doctors take their office work home.
- Some nurses, to help with staff shortage, will work continuously for 16 hours.
- Some doctors will see patients when they are off duty.

In the medical arena, we do not have barriers to error. We have barriers to good judgment and work. Therefore when we invert Reason's Swiss Cheese Model we better portray medical conditions. See Figure 7.

The Barriers to Good Performance
Barriers to good work or enhancers of reptilian influence are:
- Acute sleep loss and the later part of the graveyard shift
- Haste

43

GOOD JUDGMENT

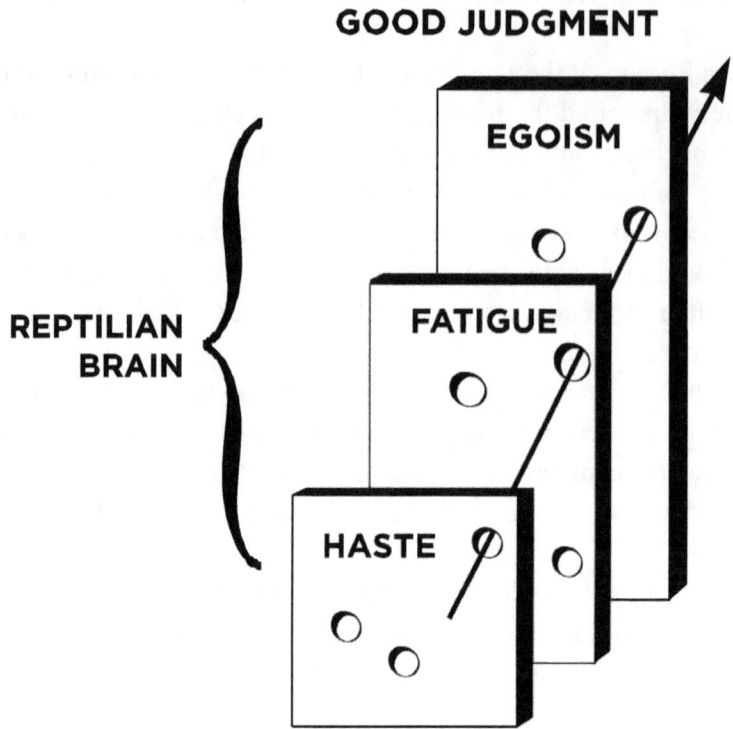

Figure 7 The Inverted Swiss Cheese Model

- Inconvenient time of consultation
- Egoism
- Acute Stress
- Chronic Stress (Burnout)

These major barriers to good performance are examined in Part II (Chapters 6-9).

CHAPTER 6

Acute Sleep Loss and the Graveyard Shift

Acute sleep loss is a cheap drunk for the physician but expensive for the patient.

I first experienced the power of acute sleep loss in 1966. I had passed Second Med, and had a high-paying summer job on Glomar IV, an oil rig, in the North Sea. After working the 12 hour night shift, I continued to work late into the morning, unloading pipes, from a supply ship to the rig. I was standing high on its upper deck, gently rocking over and back by a soft swell in the splendor of a summer's morning. When each pipe came toward me, I had to duck and guide it to rest parallel to the others. I remember a pipe coming toward me, and if it had hit me, it would have sent me to the deck below. I did not move. I remember I was too tired to care if I lived or died. The coming pipe hit an upright and was blocked in its knock-down punch. Tiredness had robbed me of the basic urge to survive.

Sleep is regulated by our reptilian brain and sleep deprivation elephants other urges.[43] Ever drive a car when sleepy? One knows that falling asleep could lead to a crash, yet one can continue to drive and nod off.

The effects of fatigue were highlighted on August 18th 1993, when a Douglas DC-8-61 crashed approximately ¼ mile from the approach end of the runway at Guantanamo Bay. This accident took place at 5 PM. It was discovered that the crew members had an acute sleep loss. They were continuously awake for 19, 21, and 23.5 hours prior to the accident.

Acute sleep loss also threatens doctors' lives. For example, "one trainee doctor had been awake for most of the weekend on call. After his duty was finished, he drove home but fell asleep at the wheel, sustaining fractures of both lower limbs in the ensuing accident."[44]

A study of interns[45] found that:

- the odds that interns will have a documented motor vehicle crash on the commute after an extended work shift were more than double the odds after a non-extended shift.
- near-miss incidents were five times as likely to occur after an extended shift as they were after a non-extended shift.

If sleep deprivation guts us of the will to live, how much sooner will it rob us of less vital functions like the will to be attentive and thorough in our consultations? In a recent study,[46] some interns still worked the traditional schedule with shifts extending 24 hours or more due to every third night call schedule. Their number of medical errors was compared to another group of interns who had limited extended work shifts and reduced number of hours worked per week. Interns made 5.6 times as many serious diagnostic errors during the traditional schedule as during the intervention (fewer hours of work and shorter extended shifts) schedule. Thirty percent of the physicians in the Ely[47] group stated that they were fatigued at the time of their erroneous decision. Fatigue was deemed one of the three causes of error by the internists in the Christensen study.[48]

Extended Sleep Deprivation and Alcohol levels

Research equates sleep deprivation to blood levels of alcohol. To provide an easily grasped index of sleep deprivation and fatigue, research has conducted tests which illustrate hours of sleep deprivation as an equivalent of blood alcohol levels.[49] In this study, forty subjects participated in two

Figure 8 Performances Comparing Blood Alcohol Levels and Sustained Wakefulness

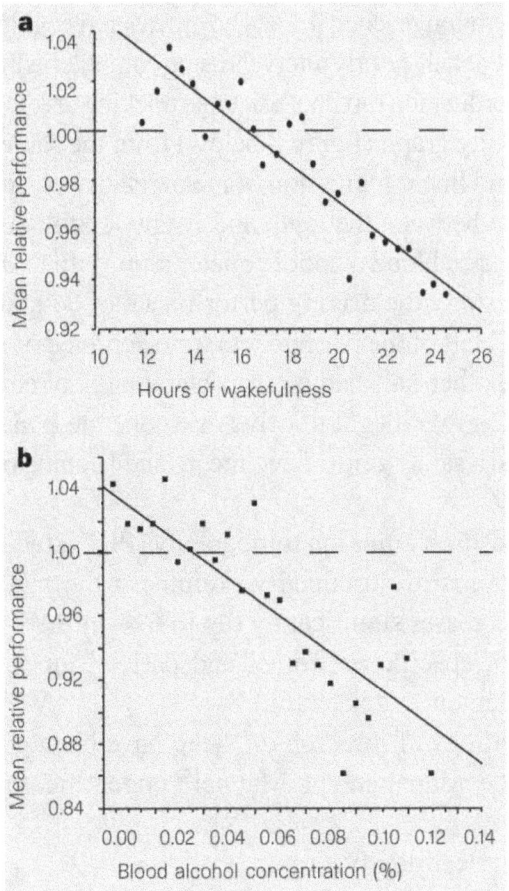

FIGURE 8 Scatter plot and linear regression of mean relative performance levels against: a, time, between the tenth and twenty-sixth hour of sustained wakefulness ($F_{1,24}$=132.9, P<0.05, R^2=0.92); and b, blood alcohol concentrations up to 0.13%, ($F_{1,24}$=54.4, P<0.05, R^2=0.69).

counter balanced experiments. In one, they were kept awake for 28 hours (from 8 until 12 the following day), and in the other, they were asked to consume 10-15 g alcohol at 30-min intervals from 8 until their mean blood alcohol concentration reached 0.1%. They measured cognitive psychomotor performance at half-hourly intervals using computer-administrated tests of hand-eye coordination (an unpredictable tracking task).

The following graph (figure 8 below) from the same article shows a scatter plot and linear regression of mean relative performance levels against: a) time between the tenth and twenty-sixth hour of sustained wakefulness and b) blood alcohol concentrations up to 0.13%.

In another study, the driving performance of 64 male participants was measured. Half of the participants were deprived of sleep the night before and the other half had a mean blood alcohol content = 0.07% (a level at which it is illegal to drive or to operate a machine).[50] Both groups revealed a safety-critical decline in lane-keeping performance in simulated traffic.

Glucose positron emission tomography (PET) studies have shown that after 24 hours of sustained wakefulness, the metabolic activity of the brain decreases significantly (up to 6% for the whole brain and up to 11% for specific prefrontal and parietal lobes, areas of self-reflection, judgment and listening).[51]

Salient findings of research on sleep have been gathered in The Crew Resource Management Manual[52] under the following three headings:
- Effects of sleep deprivation
- Sleep deprivation countermeasures
- Myths about Sleep Deprivation
- My comments are bracketed.

Effects of sleep deprivation
Sleep deprived pilots:
- are less vigilant, more willing to accept below par performance, more irritable and moody.
- have hampered inquiry, advocacy, conflict resolution, decision-making, doubting and ability to critique.

- may not easily accept an assessment of degraded performance or be able to improve their performance despite increased effort.
- become stubborn to accept criticism of their fitness. (This trait is reminiscent of the drunk refusing to relinquish the car keys).
- have impaired memory, inability to process information, and reduced mathematical skills (which are new brain activities).
- can experience micro-sleep. During a micro-sleep, a person dis- engages from reality and becomes unresponsive. They fail to respond to outside information. This event can last for a few seconds or a few minutes. (This state resembles **absence seizures**. Here the person may appear to be staring into space with or without jerking or twitching of muscles. These periods last for seconds, or even tens of seconds. Those experiencing absence seizures sometimes move from one location to another without any purpose. Sometimes they lead to periods of absence from reality, mimicking petit mal).

Sleep deprivation countermeasures from the aviation industry.

- Do not fly (work) with a sleep debt. Make this a priority over outside activities. NASA studies have shown that an individual who received 8 hours of sleep is better able to carry out pilot duties after being awake for 20 hours, than a pilot who received just 6 hours sleep.
- Pre-planning for a known sleep disruption is essential for managing alertness. Develop a regular pre-sleep routine, sleep in a comfortable environment. (Strive to have a stumble-dark, quiet room).
- Proper diet, physical conditioning, avoiding smoking and alcohol will help the body to stay healthy and be able to cope for a little longer with the effects of fatigue.
- Use caffeine sparingly during flight (work) as it may keep one awake afterward when one is trying to sleep. Water is favored to counteract caffeine's diuretic (dehydration) effects.
- If one wakes up spontaneously and cannot go back to sleep

within 15-20 minutes, or has trouble falling to sleep, get up and try again later.

- A 40-minute nap will help to rejuvenate an individual without one entering into a deep sleep, from which it is more difficult to wake.

- The aviation industry regulates the hours that pilots work.[53]

- (Other suggestions include; casino staff hours, staff change at 3 AM to overcome the impaired performance later in the traditional night shift. Also have beds available for staff to nap during night shifts).

Myths about Sleep Deprivation[54]

It is a myth that will or skill, or increased effort, or stamina, or physical conditioning, or education, or training, or experience, or professionalism, or motivation can counteract a pilot suffering the effects of acute sleep loss.

It is a myth that we can readily feel the onset of fatigue. No. Sleep can stalk and pounce on us like a cat. (I have suddenly nodded off at the wheel only to be awakened by the corrugations on the shoulder of the road).

It is a myth that one can indefinitely deny one's body of its required sleep. **The only cure for a sleep debt is sleep**. One cannot substitute this debt with anything else.

It is a myth that one can estimate one's own alertness and performance, especially if the individual has a history of flying with sleep deprivation and feels motivated enough to overcome the adverse effects.[55]

(Yet some residents and interns are sometimes scheduled to work 80-120 hours a week. The European Union is attempting to establish limits to hours of work for physicians. European doctors are resisting these proposed legislations).

50

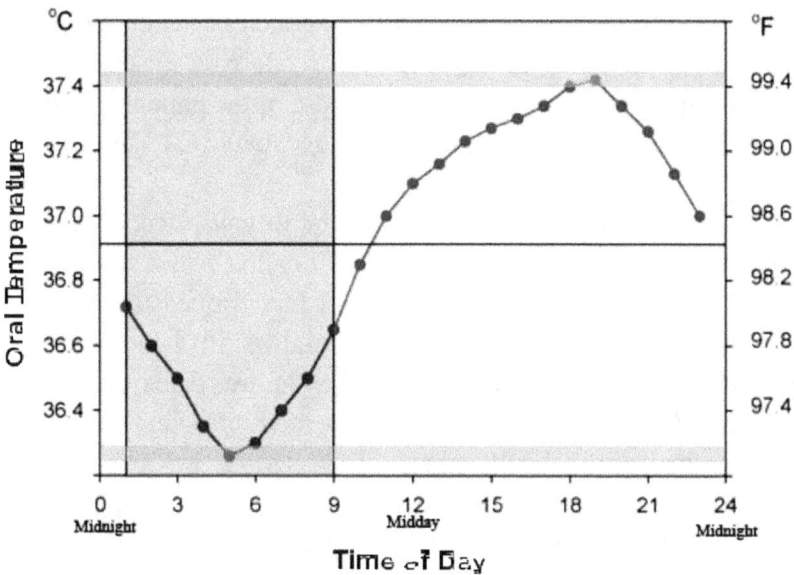

Figure 9 Body Temperature over 24 hours

The Graveyard Shift
The later part of the graveyard shift also can be a cheap drunk.

In my Emergency Department between 4 AM to 6 AM, when activity had slowed down, I recall having seen one or two nurses slumped over the counter asleep, swaddled with blankets to keep warm.[56] Our core body temperature drops 2° F between 4 AM and 6 AM[57] (Figure 9 on next page).

Our basal metabolic rates (BMR) also drop during the same period.[58] BMR is the amount of energy expended by the body while at rest.

During this same period, human performances such as logical reasoning and mental arithmetic worsen only to recover around dawn. Studies have shown that between the hours of 4 AM and 8 AM on the first night of a night shift, performance is equivalent to having a blood alcohol equal to or greater than 0.05%, a level illegal for driving or operating a machine.[59]

My own experiences of the Graveyard Shift
Later in the midnight shift I used to become more irritable. Be-

51

tween 3 AM and 6 AM, I could hear the couch in the doctor's sleep room call my name, "John, John." I craved to answer the call so much that my major goal was how I could dispose of the patients as quickly as possible. An acronym for this attitude is GOOMER: get out of my emergency room.[60]

During these midnight shifts, my irritability was accompanied by poor judgment. For example, at 3.30 AM, I called a surgeon for imagined air under the diaphragm because I had flipped the X-ray the wrong way round. During another midnight shift, I thought that a drunk was aggressive due to alcohol when he was discovered to have a sub-dural hematoma by the emergency room physician (ERP) who took over this case in the morning.

Once sitting by a patient's bedside and asking him what was the matter, I fell asleep for an hour. The nurses let me sleep. I expect they were happy to have a break from orders. When I awoke, I found that the patient had fallen asleep. I then woke the patient. Both of us felt bet- ter and I continued with my consultation. The patient's relatives were most grateful that I had taken so much time with their father.

When I was younger, I seemed more able to sustain the night shift. But as I grew older I found that 3AM to 5AM became a time if not of irrefutable sleepiness at least one when I tended to adopt a cavalier attitude. I continued to work in the emergency room until I was 58 years of age. The only way that I could safely work through the night was to sleep a few hours before the shift and also to rest for an hour between 2AM and 5AM.

Many doctors are asleep to the dangers of sleep deprivation. We would not tolerate our taxi drivers or pilots to be sleep-deprived for 20 hours and yet some physicians and nurses present to their midnight shift following 12 hours of wakefulness. Add another eight hours of work and one is over 20 hours without sleep and this is compounded by the inevitable decline in logical reasoning and mental arithmetic between 4AM and 8AM.

Summary
Acute sleep deprivation, the tasteless drunk, reduces our prefrontal

52

and parietal lobe activity, compromising our judgment, mental arithmetic and duties. It can pounce any time, night or day and anywhere: Guantanamo Bay, the hospital, the office, the car, or even at noon out of the clear blue sky of the North Sea.

CHAPTER 7

HASTE, WHEN THE CONSULTATION IS INCONVENIENT AND A PHYSICIAN'S PARABLE ABOUT TIME

When a man does what needs to be done,
He does not know the meaning of time. -Chief Dan George [61]

The following verbatim accounts of physicians ascribe hurrying as a cause of their errors. [62]

"I was in a hurry, and I just didn't stop to think about all the possibilities. I mean I know about (name of the disease), they teach that in medical school and I knew about it.... But I just didn't even think about it..... But I didn't even think about it. I was just in a hurry, you know, in a hurry to get to the next (patient)."

"...the physician was in a hurry because his partner's patient had been worked into his schedule on a busy Friday afternoon."

"Another doctor shared the perception that being chronically busy because of a large patient load had led him to be lax in supervising subordinates."

In the Ely group, 91% of the physicians felt hurried. [63] In a question- naire of Case Western Reserve School of Medicine graduates, 47% ex- pressed major dissatisfaction due to time pressures "besides the lack of leisure time, having too many patients to see in too short a time, a large case load, and too much time on call were mentioned repeatedly." [64] Thirty-five percent of Canadians think the word "rushed" describes their family physician very well. Indeed, more than three-quarters of Canadian physicians feel very rushed.[65]

Time has been called the fourth dimension in which we live. From the time we get up in the morning to the time we go to bed, most of our days are measured or ruled by time. And so it is not surprising that time towers over our practices and mistakes. We rarely credit time for our successes, but we are ready to blame it for our mistakes.

Time is everywhere, in the home, on the T.V., VCR, microwave, cell phone, computer, oven, wrist and even if you get away in your car, there's a clock there for you as well. Time is also prominently displayed in the hospital, like icons in a church.

What does the clock tell us? Or more accurately, what do we ex- perience when we look at the time? It nags, "you're late." Time rarely soothes, rarely whispers, "linger a while where you are, you are where you should be and you are doing what you should be doing. Take your time." So time, as we experience it, is not a few impartial numbers but a prod to hurry up, often a wish to escape doubting or to end the day's heavy list, and escape is one of the reptile's reflexes. Haste is not merely a glance, it is a stride, an escape to the future, corrupting new brain ac- tivities such as listening, discernment and reasoning, activities which can only take place in the present.

Looking at the time is an expression of impatience with the pres- ent and its challenges, insinuating that the present activity is not as much a priority as our future obligations. Time speculation also distracts us from our vigilance to the task at hand.

Is our vassalage to time a sign of a greater malaise within us? Or we might ask, why do we not want to be doing what we are doing? Why do we wish to be somewhere else? These questions will be addressed later under Burnout in Chapter 9.

The difference between a thorough consultation and an inadequate one may be no more than checking the vital signs, or a

56

physical sign, or asking the patient or relative five or six more questions to clarify the history, or checking for blood in the rectum, or, if the patient has a tooth infection, checking the immune status, the heart valves and his- tory for possible drug allergies. Or it might mean retaking the history and performing the examination again. The time needed to exercise due diligence and care should not be a consideration. (Many doctors will disagree because their bosses want them to see more patients in a shift. However, the patient expects the physician to be diligent. Our courts also use these same expectations implied in the patient-physic- ian contract).

Time watching can lower the patient's sense of merit, labeling the patient less deserving of our time than those following or our after- work obligations. We watch the time less when we care or are more in- terested in a patient and we watch time more when the patient annoys or challenges us.

Can we ignore time? Yes. We forget about time when we are in- volved with something we enjoy, like a past-time.[66] But can we ignore time in our offices? When I worked at The Victoria Hospital in St. Lucia, the nurses recorded the patient's respiratory and pulse rates using sand glasses, which measured one minute. I think that the doctor might well experiment by hiding all the time pieces in his or her office and use only a sand glass to measure the pulse and respiratory rates. This could be an experiment to see if we can survive without knowing what time it is.Thus we might break free of time's criticism of our present state, and become content with the present task.

Time watching is serving time. It distracts us from the task at hand, from listening to the history or the breath sounds, or appreciating what our hands are palpating. Strange as it sounds, it is only by ignoring time that we can have time for the patient we are tending.

The Time of the Consultation was Inconvenient for the Physician

> *"Things that matter most must never be at the mercy of things which matter least." -*
> **Goethe**

For me, the circumstances leading to the death of my dog a few years ago provide a poignant example of the time of consultation being inconvenient for the doctor. Guinness, our 9-year-old black Labrador bitch, began to act strange one evening. At 10 PM I examined her and concluded that she had a bowel obstruction. I called our vet and I re- lated the history of her illness together with her vital signs

These were abnormal, including increased respiratory rate and labored breathing (Kussmaul Respiration).[67] The vet informed me that she would see our dog in the morning. I said that I wanted her seen now and she replied that there was nothing she could do tonight as there was no technician available to help take an X-ray. When my dog died the following morning the vet was upset and confessed that she could have called a technician in the previous night. Had I called the vet during clinic hours, Guinness would have been treated promptly. This refusal and dishonesty is a caution to how convenience can buckle judgment, integrity, and performance.

In the Ely group, 42% of the physicians found that the time of the consultation was stressful for them, e.g., night, weekend, "off-duty" hours, or "quitting" time.[68] The following verbatim account of a physician also describes this inconvenience: *"And I can see, looking back… where you try and make it fit something less than it is to justify your course of action and plan at the time. I can see all those other pressures where everybody wants to shut down the clinic. It's been a long day, get home, get out. Do I really want to go up and do all this stuff? Do I want to have the (consultant) see him, do I want to do the blood count, and the (procedure) and mess with trying to get an IV started and all those other things that very quickly go through your mind, and you say, ' Well, I don't think the patient is that sick'."*

The pilots call this urge **go-home-itis**. At Tenerife Airport, a KLM Boeing 707 attempted to take off without clearance and crashed into a Pam Am Boeing. 583 crew and passengers were killed. It was later discovered that the KLM pilot had go-home-itis. His plane had been diverted and delayed due to a bomb at Las Palmas and he was **hurrying** home.[69]

What has quitting time to do with taxiing onto a runway or with the patient's pathology? Or "after-hours" work with a dog's strangled bowel? One has to be extra vigilant when one is seeing a patient at an inconvenient time. The reptilian influence heightens when we en- counter inconvenience. We lean away from the inconvenient toward a convenient solution. When a friend asks you about his stomach pain when you are leaving the hospital, when you are striding onto the ice or golf links, or about to go to sleep or any time that is inconvenient to you, note that your friend now is labeled a nuisance. Monitor your irritability barometer, beware of yourself. You may not be in your right mind, not fit to tend the patient, because now, things that matter most are at the mercy of things that matter least.

A Medical Parable about Time

The following is what happened to the late Dr. Orville Messenger, a thoracic surgeon when he "spent time with a patient."[70]

"Looking back on the hundreds of patients, I treated for cancer of the lung, and reflecting on the very few for whom surgery provided a real cure, I know I'd have been better spending more time with many of them at the bedside and less in the operating room.

"I do remember one special example of the value of extra time spent with a patient. One night an ambulance brought a patient from a facility that cares for elderly patients. Amos, we'll call him, was well over eighty years of age and had been a resident for many years at that home. No relatives visited him and little was known about his background. He was a deaf mute and was considered to have suffered a stroke. His only ability was to grimace in response to pain and to wave his hands in a jerky sort of

59

way.

"The note on Amos's referral sheet stated that for twenty-four hours he had vomited everything he had been given. He did look ill and was obviouslydehydrated and had a fever. His face registered pain, particularly when I pressed on his abdomen with my hand. I sat with Amos for a long while trying to sort out whether or not he needed an operation.

"What makes Amos's case special is this - while I was sitting at his bedside I began to notice what seemed like a certain repetitive pattern to his odd hand movements.[71] It dawned on me that perhaps Amos was trying to communicate. Could this be some sort of sign language? I contacted a friend who signed for a group of deaf people at our local church. After watching him, she was convinced that he was signing, but in a strange way that she could not understand. She told me that her grandmother had been deaf and had used an archaic form of hand signing that had long ago had been dropped by the deaf community. She looked up the signs somewhere, came back and tried some signs on Amos.

"It was an electrifying moment - through his pain came a smile and tears of joy that after so many years someone had finally taken the time to understand him. From that time on we could get through to Amos and he could talk to us. There were tears in my eyes, I assure you, and I look back at that experience as one of my most satisfying moments in medicine. It was my reward for spend-ing time."

CHAPTER 8

EGOISM

Man becomes free through the realization of his nothingness.
-Sartre

The reptile vigorously defends its territory for its food and prog-
eny. Likewise physicians, despite their large new brain, can emphatically
defend three territories:
- Assumptions
- Diagnoses
- Self esteem among peers and patients.

Egoism and emphasis

Here is a physician's account, from the Ely article, emphatically de-
fending his or her intellectual territory, *"All of a sudden, they were just suddenly concerned, to the point where they were really irritating me. Like, "did you
check this, did you check this?" And the mother was in between the patient and
me and wouldn't get out of the way so I could look at the patient. She wasn't doing
this on purpose, but I was really getting angry. I examined her again. I don't find
anything specific. And I'm really angry now. And by this time I'm not
listening. I'm not making the right decisions, I'm saying, "Absolutely not...."* [72]

Egoism: preserving our self-esteem

"Nothing is too good for my patient provided that it involves no
shame for me."[73]

Two accounts follow of where advocacy for our self-image trumps
advocacy for the patient. Again from the Ely Group:

"At that point, I was still in training and I wasn't completely competent when it came to technical things, I was fatigued, I was fearful of looking as incompetent as I was, so that I didn't feel that I could call on the people that I really needed to help me. I wasn't supposed to be calling. That was a sign that you were a 'wuss'"

"Because to convince these guys to drive an hour and a half to go to (name of city) to get a CT scan and then (it would) be midnight and then try to convince the physician that I thought this person needed a CT scan... uh (shakes head). ...You know, they'd say, 'Yeah, right, doc.'"

The internists in the Christensen article named pride as one of the three causes for their mistakes, one saying that pride had prevented him from readmitting a patient he had previously discharged.[74] I know of a patient who presented at 3AM with an intestinal hemorrhage. The physician did not wake the consultant; he feared the consultant's tirade. The patient did not survive.[75]

For theologians, pride motivates and directs all the other sins because it puts the creature before God. Similarly, egoism puts the physician before the patient. Theologians list offshoots of pride: disobedience, hypocrisy, strife, obstinacy, and presumption. Some of these offshoots re- semble hazardous attitudes found in the cockpit, namely, anti-authority,

machoism and invulnerability.

Egoism is a glance away from the patient to one's self-interest, and when one looks back the patient has become more of an inconvenience, an irritant. Egoism tempts to trade reality for preening our self-esteem, imagining imminent and future shames, firstly with the consultant and then along the gossip-vine to other physicians about one's ignorance or lack of competence.

The opposite of egoism is humility. Being humble means honoring the truth by submitting to it no matter how embarrassing it might be. Humility makes doubting and broadcasting that doubt easier; egoism makes it harder. I was often reluctant to consult because it would reveal my ignorance. It takes gumption and humility to consult when it reveals our ignorance and/or incompetence. It requires no courage to consult when it broadcasts our clinical acumen.

C. S. Lewis wrote that humility is a great relief because it frees us from being ourselves.[76] The tyrant that we need to escape is our self-image. Preserving our self-image is a basic instinct which we need to overcome in order to acknowledge and to communicate our doubts, ignorance or incompetence to a sometimes unwelcoming if not hostile self or an equally unwelcoming if not hostile colleague.

C.S. Lewis describes a humble man as one who is interested in the other person. "Probably all you will think about him is that he seemed a cheerful, intelligent chap who took a real interest in what you said to him. He will not be thinking about humility. He will not be thinking about himself at all. If anyone would like to acquire humility, I can, I think, tell him the first step. The first step is to realize that one is proud."[77]

There is a misconception that humility means groveling, acquiescing to others, a Quisling.[78] It is the egoists who grovel, who acquiesce, to their self-image and self-interest. The humble person is empowered to advocate, to speak truth to power; the egoist, when threatened, slinks away, blending with the foliage of the status quo.

Can we gauge the intensity of this love affair with ourselves? This insight is difficult if not impossible. Some clues might present themselves. When we arrive at our work station, do we look at the on-call list to check the receptivity of the consultants for this shift? Do we prefer to call one consultant more than another? Do we change the story depending on the consultant we address? By contrast, the humble will not weigh the receptivity of one consultant against another and will not waver regardless of who the on-duty consultant is, looking on "friend and foe" with an equal eye, an advanced counter-reptilian response. We can also check our poise for reptilian characteristics, especially emphatic expressions. (Table 1, Chapter 3) A reliable compass in this reptilian fog is the question, "Would I like to be treated as I am treating this patient?"

Can we suppress the ego? No, but we can monitor it, by asking ourselves, "who does this thought, diagnosis or action serve, the patient or me?"

Gumption, to speak the unflattering truth to power, is not dependent on physical prowess. I have seen a frail small nurse advocate on behalf of her patient to an imposing intimidating doctor. I have also seen a big male physician buckle before the same consultant.[79] Sartre reminds us one becomes free through the realization of one's nothingness.

Egoism pretends all that we are; humility acknowledges all that we are not.[80] Egoism is hypocritical, a scam to avoid shame, a betrayal of the patient's trust. Humility prioritizes the patient, and empowers us to speak the whole truth to the tyrant within and the bully without.

CHAPTER 9

ACUTE STRESS, CHRONIC STRESS AND BURNOUT

ACUTE STRESS

"I'm a Professional- This won't happen to me!"
-Anthony Grasha

Pilots believe that if our stress level is very high, we operate at low levels of situational awareness.[81] For example, a pilot landed twice with gear landing up because his wife had a threatened miscarriage. I experienced this low level of situational awareness when I drove through the blinking pedestrian lights, at that moment I was preoccupied by my patient who had died from the volvulus.

Severe stress, be it guilt, grief or joy, buckles our mental axle, frequently veering us back toward the recent big event, away from the task at hand. After a stressful event it takes time to balance our alignment, to focus on the task at hand. Another example; one week after a pharmacist had buried his wife, he dispensed an adult dose of a narcotic for an 18-month-old child. The pharmacist's boss allowed him only a week off work for bereavement.[82]

The Christensen group of physicians[83] claimed that there is cynicism about the tendency of colleagues to minimize a physician's mistake. These same physicians often feel isolated and sometimes fail to share their mistakes or concerns with their colleagues or even their spouses. Another author referred to a "conspiracy of silence,"[84] this soli- tary shouldering of one's mistake is a sign of how physicians neglect themselves and neglect to seek perspective and help from colleagues.

Chronic Stress

"Self-love, my liege, is not so vile a sin as self-neglecting."
-King Henry V (Act 2 Scene 4)

Chronic stress is not as dramatic as acute stress. Yet the aviation in- dustry claims that chronic stress impairs good judgment more than acute stress. The aviation industry also claims that "Too much stress will de- tract from the pilot's ability to reason and function, by eroding inquiry, advocacy, conflict resolution, decision making and critiquing."[85] The authors of the Ely article reported that "many participants disclosed embarrassing details about their emotional states at the time of the error."[86]

What is the prevalence of chronic stress among physicians?

The prevalence of Chronic Stress among physicians

In 2003, the Canadian Medical Association hoped to measure the degree of job stress and burnout among physicians. It mailed a Profes- sional Stress and Burnout questionnaire to 8,172 members. The au- thors concluded that 46% of the 2,250 Canadian physicians who responded to the questionnaire were in the advanced stages of burnout.[87] Female physicians were 60% more likely to suffer burnout. Another study reported that at least 44% of physicians specializing in infectious diseases suffered burnout.[88]

How serious can burnout be? In the worst cases, burnout can be the last ledge to the big drop. The United States loses the equivalent of graduates from seven entire medical schools (approximately 700 physicians) per year due to alcoholism, drug addiction and suicide.[89] Drug addiction may be between 30 and 100 times more common among physicians than in the general population.[90] Physicians are more likely to have had 10 or more visits to a psychiatrist than controls.[91] The suicide rate of physicians is two to eight times that of the general population.[92-93]

Sadly, the effects of stress are already evident in postgraduate training and even in medical students. Suicides are second in number only to accidents as the cause of death among medical students,[94] and drug abuse is common among medical students.[95-96]

Two studies have shown that about one third of interns have frequent episodes of emotional distress or depression,[97-98] and a quarter of these interns have suicidal ideation.[99] This is a sad indictment on how much we have neglected our present and future physicians. Many physician associations now provide interventions and preventative programs. See footnote No 113 for examples.

Burnout and stress are not synonymous. Burnout is a state of being. Stress, on the other hand, is a neutral event which produces energy and urgency in the non-burnout person, but a sense of helplessness and despair in the person who is suffering burnout.

What is Burnout?

Burnout is a syndrome which includes one or more of the following three states:
- Emotional exhaustion;
- Depersonalization;
- Low sense of personal accomplishment.

These first two states are more common among physicians than the third.[100]

The Burnout Syndrome

Emotional exhaustion is compassion fatigue. It can be described as a failure of the mental "muscle" that pumps forth care for our patients, and families. One teacher, who suffered burnout, described it to me as "plodding on empty in Fundy mud up to my knees. I've had it

I can take no more. Just leave me alone."

At work, we feel like handing the patient a phone and saying "call someone who cares." We find that everything and everyone is getting on our nerves. Contact with others drains us and we often ask, "What are we doing, here?" We react to delays in the office or operating room as if they are major crises. We lack what Pirsig called "psychic gasoline."[101]

With ongoing stresses, our "caring muscle" weakens, and can flat-line. We become "wounded healers."[102] Then we abandon hope that our work or our lives can improve. Inexorably, we circle the drain of despair and apathy.

Depersonalization is a withdrawal from others, no longer enjoying our friends and family whose company we used to enjoy, going through the motions like a robot. It is a crisis of our worth as a person. To wade through the day, we employ emotion-saving techniques, such as avoiding eye contact, becoming brusque, blunt and even callous. Because doctors are advised not to allow themselves to feel too much sympathy or sadness, we often deny our own emotions and some physicians may shut down emotionally. McCue, writing in the New England Journal of Medicine, values emotional stability: *"... placing the patient's interests before those of the physician, and considering all the ramifications of a therapeutic or diagnostic intervention (cost benefit analysis) require concentration by a physician who enjoys the work and brings to it an emotional stability derived from his or her personal life."*[103]

Personal Achievement is diminished. We can find little joy in medicine. We don't feel we make a difference anymore. We enter a hell where we begin to abandon hope that we can ever make a difference. We question the worth of our work and finally it becomes a crisis of our worth as a physician.

Burnout Neurobiology: Brain Derived Neurotrophic Factor
Burnout is now being better understood. Parts of the adult brain retain the ability to grow new neurons from neural stem cells in a process known as neurogenesis. Brain derived neurotrophic factor (BDNF) is

one of the chemicals that stimulates and controls this neurogenesis and is thought to contribute to the neurobiology of burnout syndrome. In one study, 37 clinically diagnosed burnout participants were compared to 35 healthy controls in terms of BDNF levels. They found lowered levels of serum BDNF in the burnout group as compared to that of the healthy controls.[104] BDNF is active in the hippocampus, cortex, and basal forebrain, areas vital to learning, memory, and higher thinking. Perhaps Pirsig's psychic gasoline can be named *brain derived neurotrophic factor.*

The effects of burnout, therefore, can be understood as expressions of the reptilian brain,[105] a reptilian brain untrammeled by the now enfeebled centers of higher thinking.

Burnout also impairs our ability to appreciate doubt. The increased irritability that signals doubt is masked by the heightened irritability which often accompanies burnout.

When does burnout occur?
"Too much of a sacrifice can make a stone of the heart." - Yeats[106]

According to Wright, burnout is a problem born of good intentions to attempt to reach unrealistic goals, when the high effort does not yield the expected results, and the physician ends up depleting his or her energy and losing touch with themselves and others.[107] Burnout occurs when demands exceed reserves.[108] Certainly for many physicians, life seems an unending series of demands at work and at home.

At work, these demands include more patients, more complications, more paperwork, more committees, and a monthly avalanche of journals to read. Then there are unrelenting frustrations, such as difficulties admitting patients to hospital, getting diagnostic tests and consultations in a timely manner. Moreover, there are the unavoidable frustrations of what Dr. Groves called "The Insatiable Dependency of the Hateful Patient."[109] Not infrequently there arises a feeling of "helplessness in the healer."[110] The CMA also noted that some physicians – especially women, minorities or those who practice in remote or underserved areas – have extra stressors.[111]

And when we are at work, we think that we should be at home, and when we are at home we often think about our work.

Our homes can be stressful. The demands of work frustrate family plans. When our friends are free on week-ends and holidays, physicians and nurses are often working. This is also often a source of conflict between spouses.

On-call duties and shift work invade our homes and scramble our circadian rhythms. Children balk at their homework, squabble and rebel and may have chronic serious disabilities. And the stay-at-home spouse, often needs to get out and socialize. By contrast, the physician might need tranquility to recharge for the next day's work.

Many who suffer burnout lack boundaries on their time, and sometimes they lack the ability or the courage to say "no." I know of specialists who work long hours and take their work home with them where they read E.C.G.s or E.E.G.s or complete their paper-work late into the evening. What physician, upon hearing one of their patients reveal such long hours of work, would not prescribe shorter hours of work and more relaxation? Yet we are blind to our accumulating stresses, believing that we can, without diastole, push ourselves, without consequences. The likelihood of burnout appears to increase by 10% for each extra hour of work beyond 40 hours per week.[112] About 24% of Canadian physicians work 60-79 hours a week, excluding calls.[113] We ignore the pleas of our families and friends to work less.

Self-care is not part of the physician's professional training and typically is low on a physician's list of priorities. According to a survey of graduates of Johns Hopkins School of Medicine, approximately one third of physicians do not have a doctor themselves.[114] Physicians deal with other people's problems all day, but they're the least likely to raise their own personal problems. We should not neglect but rather tend the wounded healer.

How do we know if we are suffering burnout?

There are many Internet links which have questionnaires to answer this question.[115]

Dr. Gautam in her book "Irondoc" lists five early warning signs

70

for burnout:[116]
- Increased physical problems or illnesses.
- Increased problems with relationships.
- Increased negative thoughts and feelings, about things and people that one previously enjoyed.
- Increased unhealthy behaviors.
- Inability to continue to push ourselves.

Preventing and treating burnout

There are many associations[117] which have programs to assist physicians with stress in their lives and work. Dr. Gautam's book, "Irondoc", outlines a practical program to help the physician deal with stresses. It is a short read, and her 20 training tips should be revisited regularly by a physician throughout his or her life.[118] One of her tips, I found especially poignant, namely, "Remember the 90:10 Rule." Dr. Gautam writes, "In any situation in which you feel stress and think that you are over-reacting, you probably are. Remember, 90% of your reaction is from the past, the Historian. Only 10% of your reaction is due to the situation you are currently dealing with."

I would like to mention two other sources for coping with stress:
- Viktor Frankl's method from his book, "Man's Search for Meaning."[119]
- A Mindfulness-based Stress Reduction Program for Nurses.[120]

Dr. Viktor Frankl's reflections on stress
"We are all heirs to stresses.
How we handle them is our choice." -Viktor Frankl

Viktor Frankl, a Jewish Viennese psychiatrist, was a prisoner for three years in Nazi death camps. He spent the last of these three years in Auschwitz. Yet under such depraved, cruel and evil conditions, Viktor Frankl found that one could lessen these stresses and scramble a meaning to life. He used these techniques.
- Distance Transposition for Objectivity
- Enjoyment

- Humor
- The Belief in One's Freedom to Respond.

Distance Transposition for Objectivity

Frankl describes how he discovered the value of transposition.[121]

"Almost in tears from pain (I had terrible sores on my feet from wearing torn shoes), I limped a few kilometres with our long column of men from the camp to our work site. Very cold bitter winds struck us. I kept thinking of the endless little problems of our miserable life. What would there be to eat tonight? If a piece of sausage came as an extra ration, should I exchange for a piece of bread? Should I trade my last cigarette, which was left from a bonus I received a fortnight ago, for a bowl of soup? How should I get a piece of wire to replace the one that served as one of my shoelaces? Would I get to work in time to join my usual work party or would I have to join another, which might have a brutal foreman?

I became disgusted with the state of affairs which compelled me, daily and hourly, to think of only such trivial things. Imagine how I felt? Then by the hammer of will I forced my thoughts to turn to another subject. Suddenly, I saw myself standing on the platform of a well-lit, warm and pleasant lecture room. In front of me sat an attentive audience on comfortable seats. I was giving a lecture on the psychology of the concentration camp! All that oppressed me at that moment became objective, seen and described from the remote viewpoint of science. By this method I succeeded somehow in rising above the situation, above the sufferings of the moment, and I observed them as if they were already in the past. Both I and my troubles became the object of an interesting psychoscientific study undertaken by myself."[122]

The author has found this ability to transpose himself to a few weeks into the future weakened his present reptilian pressures. It also helped him focus more on the patient's needs.[123]

Enjoyment

"I strove to enjoy the small things that made one happy, for example: being at the head of the line, working in the factories or in a sheltered room and glad of the time to delouse before going to bed." A man once criticized to me Frankl's approach to life as being Pollyanna. Thich Nhat Hanh's[124] remark lends support to Frankl, "If you are not enjoying washing the dishes, you probably haven't enjoyed the meal."[125]

Humor

Humor is a new brain activity. Frankl wrote, "The attempt to develop a sense of humor is a trick learned while mastering the art of living. They'd dream of a dinner in the future and asking the hostess to ladle the soup from the bottom." When the physician or the nurse is encountering a hateful patient, one can take solace that one is not married to the patient, that this encounter is not a terminal state, it too will pass.

We now know that laughter releases endorphins which lower levels of stress hormones and also lowers the blood pressure.

The Belief in one's Freedom to Respond

According to Frankl, "The captors could take everything away from us but our freedom to respond."(Frankl's experiences of this freedom to respond are recounted in Chapter 2). We help create our own feeling of being un-free. We can choose to be hot reactors or not, to race through the fading orange traffic lights or relaxing, to drum our fingers impatiently at the red lights, to interrupt patients and shepherd them to- ward our agenda or choose to be content with the present. The feeling of lack of perceived control (un-free) is the highest predictor of burnout.[126]

Sartre claimed, "choice is one thing from which there is no escape."[127] The doctor can never escape choice between being rushed, and not; between being thorough and slack; between being calm and irritated; between being humorless and humorous; between doubt and certainty; between labeling and being non-judgmental; between being gracious and rude; in essence, between being reflective and reptilian.

Three hundred years before Frankl, another prisoner, Richard Lovelace, wrote of freedom's possibility in *To Althea, from Prison.*

> Stone walls do not a prison make
> Nor iron bars a cage.[128]

Another strategy for coping with stress

A Mindfulness-based Stress Reduction Program for Nurses

Nurses also are at high risk of chronic stress and burnout. A report on nurses from five countries shows that 40% of hospital nurses have burnout levels that exceed the norms for health workers.[129] At Lehigh Valley Hospital and Health Network, (LVHHN), Allentown, Pennsylvania, an 8-week Mindfulness-based Stress Reduction Program (MBSR), based on the University of Massachusetts Medical Center program created by Jon-Kabat-Zinn,[130] was offered to nurse professionals.[131] During this program, 27 volunteers attended classes for two hours a week for eight weeks. They also practiced self-care (mindfulness techniques) for 30 minutes on the other six days of the week.

The authors conclude that MBSR is an effective strategy for reducing burnout.[132] Qualitative data analysis were also recounted.[133] For example, one participant stated, "I've learned to do one day at a time, one duty at a time, one thing at a time." Another stated, "I used to stand by the microwave, impatient that the food wasn't cooking fast enough. Now, I can step back when I start to do that, laugh, and then slow down."

What is mindfulness? Kabat-Zinn describes mindfulness as "conscious moment-to-moment awareness, cultivated by systematically paying attention, on purpose, a state in which one is highly focused on the reality of the present moment, accepting and acknowledging it, without getting caught up in thoughts that are about the situation or emotional reactions to the situation."[134] Mindfulness does not create the absence of negative thoughts and emotions; rather, with mindfulness practice, one can be less caught up in them. The key to mindfulness is not simply attention. More importantly, it is how one attends. The intention one brings to attention is crucial. The attention must embody impartiality, acceptance of self and others, and patience. Mindfulness is a lifelong endeavor.[135] For more on the techniques of Mindfulness see Kabat-Zinn's book, *Full Catastrophe Living*.

In the traffic of work, moments of mindfulness are "road-side rests" of reduced or little stress. Through the hours and days, these calmers add to our reserves to reflect on the patient's condition.[136]

In the compelling article "Happiness is the frequency, not the intensity, of positive versus negative affect,"[137] the authors claim that "the frequency of positive versus negative affect is at the core of a construct we can label happiness or affective well-being."

In the calculus of stress, it is the proportion of positive to negative emotions that determines the wealth or poverty of our well-being. The more positive thoughts we have banked, the more we can give. One nurse described the bankruptcy of burnout, "One can't give from an empty basket." [138]

PART III

CHAPTER

10

FOUR VARIATIONS ON THE THEME OF DIAGNOSIS.

Croskerry remarked that misdiagnosis is accompanied by more frequent serious consequences than any other type of error in medicine.[139] Diagnosing, therefore, claims pointed attention.

Variation I
Diagnosis for Data: A Dangerous Trade

Henri Bergson, in his Introduction to Metaphysics, claims that when we exchange data for a concept, we often exchange gold coins for small change.[140] Similarly the patient presents the physician with the gold coins of data (symptoms and physical signs of his or her disease). The diagnosis is a naming, a concept, and may also be small change. What the patient receives in return might be an invention more than a discovery.

Bergson identifies snares to clear thinking: they resemble expressions of the Reptilian Brain. He warned that:[141]

- The mind craves simplicity, fixity. It seeks to reduce effort (**Convenience**)
- The concept (for the physician, a diagnosis) might be an invention not a discovery, (**Hurry**)

- The normal work of the intellect is far from being detached. We do not aim at knowledge for the sake of knowledge but in order to take sides, to draw profits, in short to satisfy our self-interest, **(Egoism)**

- Thinking usually consists of fitting concepts to data and not data to concepts.[142] Hence we try to fit a concept to data - to ask ourselves what we can do with the concept, not what the data can do for us. In other words, it is more natural for us to trawl with a net of diagnoses rather than gather and follow the symptoms and signs and see where they will lead.[143] **(Ready to Name to Diagnose, Convenience)**

In repudiating facility, Bergson endorses new brain activity.

- He claimed that intelligence is the power to ask questions of oneself. The master attitude, he says, is to challenge one's theory without any external prompt. The physician should challenge himself or herself rather than waiting for prompting from other staff, the patient or their relatives. **(To doubt, to self-reflect)**

- Bergson also recommended a certain manner of thinking which courts difficulty. (Dr. Chisholm had "courted difficulty" when he returned four times to see his patient). Bergson valued effort above everything else. **(Inconvenience).** He claimed that *the lack of effort is the clarity that many seek.*[144] We prefer the convenient to the inconvenient. Many of our errors stem from avoiding the inconvenience of an extra few questions to clarify the history and to perform the indicated clinical tests.

Variation II
A Distant View of Climbing the Devil's Ladder toward the Diagnosis

So when did you ever make a voyage of examining your own opinion? -Epictetus

Below, I have adapted Koestler's diagram (Figure 10) to illustrate

Chisholm's returns to his patient.[145] HP represents Chisholm's initial history and physical examination of his patient. D1 represents his first diagnosis. Just as Koestler explained the history of science as successful retreats from blind alleys, Dr. Chisholm had to retreat several times to arrive at the correct diagnosis.

To undo the diagnosis, one has to first acknowledge doubt. To do this we have to be patient with the process and be humble with or sus-

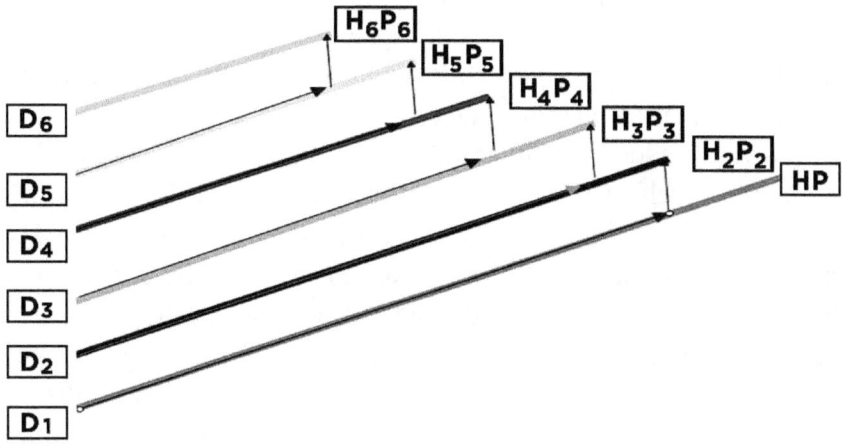

Figure 10 Undoing and Redoing in the Evolution of Diagnoses

picious of our conclusions. The more we undo the tentative diagnosis or diagnoses (D_2, D_3, etc.), the more we are willing to gather (H_2P_2, H_3P_3, etc.) and appreciate conflicting data, and the closer we approach reality.

A diagnosis is a naming activity. Naming demands little effort (depicted in the diagram as going downhill). While naming is a new brain activity, the readiness to bite on and devour a diagnosis is a reptilian urge, motivated by instant achievement and the reward of finality. By contrast, to un-name, to un-do what we have created, is more difficult, it is a retracing of one's steps uphill to potter around in the nettles of uncertainty and humility. This takes gumption. We don't have one un-prefixed synonym for un-naming. By contrast, naming has several un-prefixed synonyms. Even our verbs, the muscles of our language, are more biased toward naming than un-naming.

Devil's Ladder is a thousand-foot steep part of a route on Carrauntoohil, Ireland. When I was climbing the Devil's Ladder, my brother-in-law said that retracing to get a better approach seemed to both of us a big inconvenience. To an observer, a mile or two away, he said, it does not seem inconvenient. With this distant perspective, sub- sequent retreats on the ascent of the Devil's Ladder seemed less in- convenient to me. Similarly, physicians can obtain a distant perspective to un-naming if we can imagine ourselves three months into the future looking back at this moment of doubting. When we look back at any of our re-tracings of a few weeks ago, we wonder why we were so inconvenienced by the un-naming, why we were so impatient?

Frankl showed the benefit of the perspective afforded by viewing the present from three months into the future. Recall Frankl's Distance Transposition for Objectivity in Chapter 9.

The physician seems busy at the moment, yet looking back over our previous work we don't seem to be able to recreate the same frenetic sensation of busyness. By being aware of the rush as it happens and by then developing the three-months-in-the-future perspective of this busy situation, we can better appreciate the triviality of the cause for this haste, compared to the worth of our work.

This transposition for objectivity also enables one to follow Frankl's Categorical Imperative: *"Live as if you were living already for the second time*

and as if you had acted the first time as wrongly as you are about to act now! "[146]
Frankl believed that there was nothing which would stimulate one's
sense of responsibility[147] more than this maxim, which invites one to
imagine first that the present is past and, second, that the past may be
amended. For the physician, a contemplated omission in examination
could be imagined with its possible consequences, but still we have the
option to correct this omission now without incurring its possible
harmful results.

Variation III
When is a Diagnosis a No Brainer?

Is the diagnosis only a symptom or a sign of something else?
   We sometimes arrive at a diagnosis which later is discovered to
have been only a sign or symptom of the true underlying disease. In
Cronin's case study, Bramwell's not insignificant diagnosis of acute
homicidal mania turned out to be merely a symptom of myxoedema.
   We assume that corneal abrasions were due either due to infection
or trauma. Yet, when any pack of symptoms is shuffled, a joker can
turn up. The following article from the Lancet, "Just another corneal
abrasion?" reveals such a joker.[148]

   "A 67-year-old woman came to the ophthalmic emergency department in
   August 2000, complaining of a sore, red, right eye. She had no history of trauma
   and no previous problems with her eyes. On examination, her visual acuity was
   6/6 in the right eye, and 6/9 in the left eye. Slit lamp examination showed a
   right-sided corneal abrasion. Patients with corneal abrasions usually are uncom-
   fortable and photophobic. However, this patient did not seem particularly both-
   ered, so we tested her corneal sensation and found that it was reduced in the right
   eye. Her face was slightly asymmetrical with ptosis of the right upper eyelid. She
   had reduced sensation over the ophthalmic and maxillary divisions of her right
   trigeminal nerve, and anisocoria; the right pupil was 3mm larger than the left
   pupil. There was no afferent papillary defects and the optic discs looked normal.
   The rest of her cranial nerves were functioning normally. We questioned the
   patient in more detail about her medical history. For the past 15 years she had
   complained

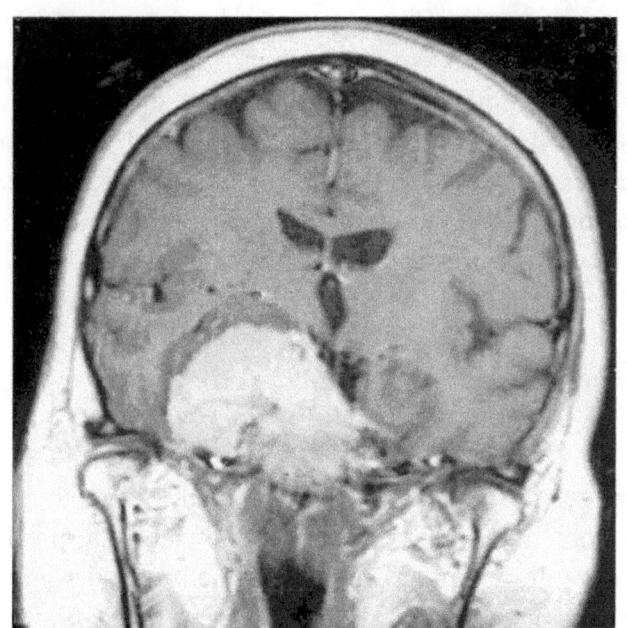

Right-sided parasellar meningioma

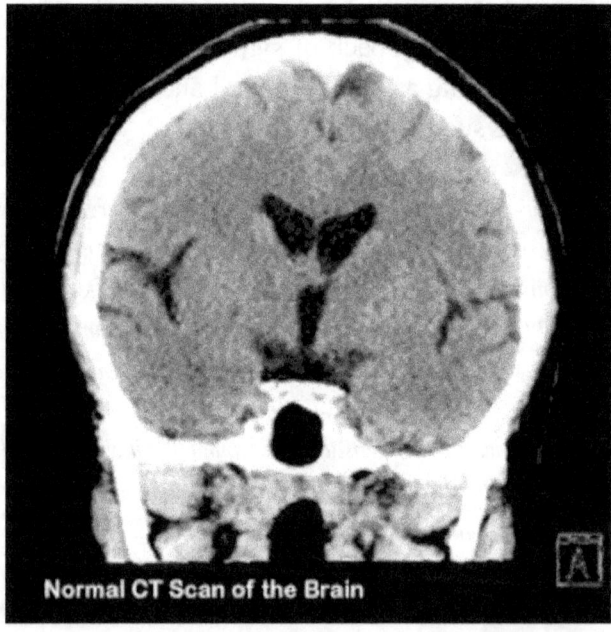

Normal CT Scan of the Brain

Figure 11 Two CT Scans of the Brain: First one (above) shows right-sided parasellar meningioma and second (below) CT Scan of a Normal Brain

of numbness and stiffness on the right side of her face. This had, after some time, been diagnosed as right trigeminal neuralgia. Over the previous 2-3 years friends had mentioned a slight drooping of the right side of her face. She had had no medical tests or treatment.

Cerebral magnetic resonance imaging with gadolinium contrast showed a large space-occupying lesion involving the right stella, cavernous sinus, and the cerebellopontine angle, probably a meningioma, arising from the petrous apex or peri-stellar region (see Figure 10). The patient was urgently referred to the neurosurgeons who decided to debulk the tumour. Following surgery, and histological confirmation of a meningioma, the patient developed a complete third nerve palsy.....

....Our patient had a partial third nerve palsy, with ipsilateral ptosis and myosis,[149] and may have had symptoms from her meningioma for over 15 years, which may have been attributed to trigeminal neuralgia. It is important to take a thorough history and not dismiss persistent, albeit minor, symptoms. We suggest that when no clear cause for a corneal abrasion is found, both the facial and the skin sensation should be checked. Now and again, there may be more than meets the eye!"

Here the authors urge us to ask why the patient has a corneal abrasion. Similarly, Dr. Manson had also asked questions: "Why, why", he kept asking "why should Hughes talk like this?" Supposing the man had gone out of his mind, what was the cause of it all? He had always been a happy, contented man - no worries, easygoing, amicable. Why, without apparent reason, had he changed to this? A child presenting with a fracture or bruises may evoke the question "Could this be child abuse?" Another way of asking this question is, "What else could this be?"[150]

The other vital question is "What else could make this diagnosis worse?"

A woman brought her nephew who had a dog bite to an emergency department. The physician checked the tetanus immunization status and cleaned the wound and discharged the patient. The aunt returned twenty hours later and said that her nephew did not seem well. Another physician examined the boy and the wound and discharged the boy. The boy died within two days. It was discovered that the boy was immunosuppressed because his spleen had been removed.

There are two kinds of questions: simple questions and problems. A simple question is readily answered, like what is the number of this page you are reading? Then there are complex questions like, when is a diagnosis a no-brainer or am I more attached to my reptilian brain now? Problems take time to answer. There are two kinds of medical questions for the medical diagnostician; the simple and the complex. It can be argued that only the complex exist for the medical physician. Why? Because it takes time to answer these two questions;

- What else could this be? For example, is this corneal abrasion, infective, traumatic or due to a neurological deficit?

- What could make this condition more complicated? For example, in the patient presenting with infection, one should also look for cardiac valvular disease and immunosuppression.

Therefore all medical questions are problems since it takes time to discover whether a case is a problem or not. The only exception is when the physician's knowledge (like the family physician) of the patient's medical history and the symptoms and signs are pathognomonic.[151] Diagnostic no-brainers are rarer than imagined. It is difficult to see the hook beneath the bait.

Also we must ask ourselves whether our diagnosis is merely a symptom or a sign of something more serious. The corneal abrasion was a sign and symptom of meningioma; acute psychosis for myxoedema and a fractured humerus in a toddler or bruises may be a sign of child abuse.

Variation IV

Clearing a Taoist Space for Making the Diagnosis

What is in your Center?

Dr. Croskerry,[152] in his seminal article, "Avoiding Pitfalls in Emergency Medicine" depicts how the emergency physician is surrounded with sources of information[153] (Figure 12). The emergency physician may be tending four or more patients at any one time. Also, interruptions are unrelenting and numerous.

Data Surrounds

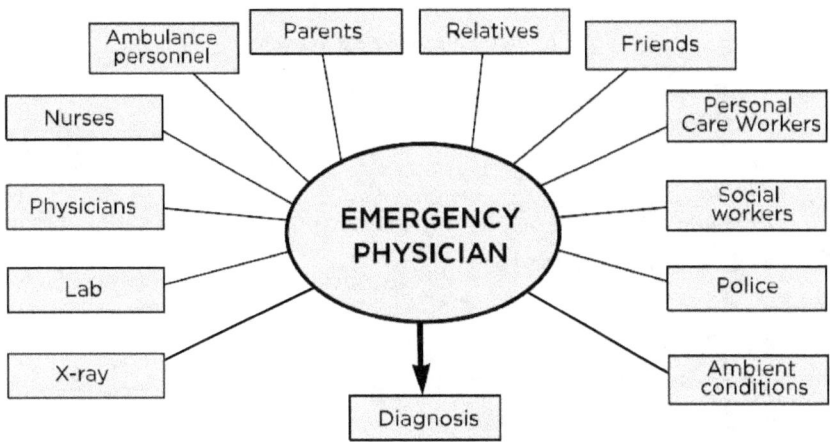

The multiple sources of both noise and useful information that may influence the emergency physician's processing of important signals.

Figure 12 Data Surrounds

Lao Tzu's Wheel

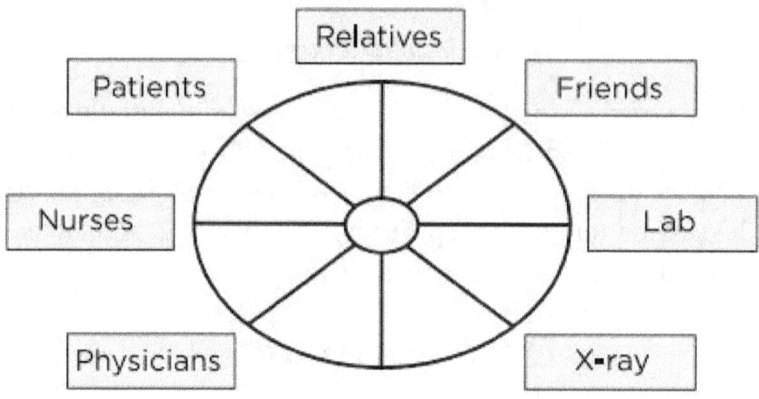

Figure 13 Lao Tzu's Wheel

One can convert Dr. Croskerry's diagram to LaoTzu's wheel from the Tao Te Ching. (Figure 13)

Lao Tzu writes of the wheel:
"Thirty spokes will converge
In the hub of a wheel;
But the use of the cart
Will depend on the part
Of the hub that is void." [154]

Unless the hub of our mind is uncluttered, it will not be able to rotate the options around. Our center may be void when we are free of reptilian influences such as desire,[155] agenda, imperatives of time, fatigue and egoism. We need our center to be clear, to search for challenging data, to welcome them, to be vigilant to the task at hand, to ask what else this could be, what else could make this worse, and would I like to be treated as I am treating now?

PART IV: LISTENING

CHAPTER 11

The Difficult Art of Listening to what one Doesn't Want to Hear

The more we listen, the more we learn.

Patients will tell you what is wrong with them, if you let them.
-Dr. Maurice Dubois

Physicians spend much of their lives taking histories from their patients. Yet despite this almost daily practice, physicians sometimes do not listen to their patients. In the Ely group, 21% of physicians did not take an adequate history or did not listen well to the history.[156]

In another study, "Clinical Hypocompetence: the Interview," the authors had observed more than 300 clinical interviews (complete or comprehensive history-taking and physical examinations) and many hundred brief interactions.[157] They observed their house staff, students and some attending staff physicians. The authors wrote, "to our surprise, all did not seem as it should be. Physicians at all levels who had previously been thought quite competent appeared defective in their interactions with patients."

The authors classify the defects in the interviews into five major syndromes.[158] They also claim that these syndromes are disorders of physicians and their processes, not of patients. The last of these syndromes they call The High Control Style- "My doctor doesn't listen."

They give a verbatim example:

Dr. X: "Hello, I'm Dr. X; are you Mrs. Y?"
Patient Y: "Yes, I'm glad to know you."
Dr: "What sorts of troubles have you been having?"
Patient Y: "I've been going downhill for two years. Nothing seems to be working right."
Dr. X; "What is the worst part?"
Patient Y: "My legs, I have constant pain in my legs. It's gotten so bad I can't sleep."
Dr. X: "What about your breathing?"
Patient Y: "Oh, that's all right. I can breathe fine. I just hurt so bad in my legs."
Dr. X: "Are you still smoking?"
Patient Y: "Yes, with this pain I've go'en back to my cigarettes for relief. But I'm down to half a pack or so a day."
Dr. X: "Are you having pains in your chest?"
Patient Y: "No."
Dr. X: "How about your cough?"
Patient Y: "No. I hardly ever cough."
Dr. X: "How much are you actually able to do?"
Patient Y: "Well, I was able to do everything until about 2 years ago, but now I can hardly walk half a block."
Dr. X: "Why is that?"
Patient Y: "My Legs. They hurt."
Dr. X: "Do they swell up?"
Patient Y: ""Well, they've been a bit swollen the last 2 or 3 weeks but the pain is there whether they swell or not."
Dr. X: "All right, I want to ask you some things about your medical history now."

Regarding this interview, the authors commented:

"The interviewer was symptom oriented. He even made an effort to elicit a chief complaint. Unfortunately he had been forewarned of a diagnosis of severe chronic lung disease, and indeed the patient appeared a bit cyanotic. It is understandable that he wanted to know about the respiratory system. However he was never able to hear the patient's story about the leg pain. During the interview the doctor tended to talk more and more, the patient less and less."

The authors also commented, "Frequently the patient seemed lim- ited to yes/no answers.[159] The interviewer needs to use phrases such as, 'Tell me about it.' Most important, he or she needs to realize that the patient's job is to tell his or her story and the physician's job is to listen..." The authors continued, "Silence, general requests, facilitation, and open-ended questions are more helpful than direct questions in developing the patient's story."

In the Crew Resource Manual in the Chapter titled: "the World's Worst Air Disaster-Tenerife, 1977," half of the headings are devoted to listening.[160] In that chapter, the manual distinguishes between active listening and its opposite. They list what active listening is not:
- passive or token, (not vigilant to what is being said)
- agreement or disagreement
- judgmental or critical of others, not critical of the listener
- argumentative, (self-asserting).

Active Listening
The aviation industry says that **active listening** is the genuine de-sire to understand another's perception and express and understand what another person has said. They describe the effective listeners in the cockpit as:
- Caring
- Trustworthy with integrity
- Accepting
- Willing to let one talk. They encourage others to speak, by being relaxed and looking toward the speaker.
- Focusing on thoughts and feelings
- Constructive and focusing on the problem, not the blame.
- Able to paraphrase. (When the physician paraphrases the patient's history it shows encouragement and also verifies accuracy of under-standing with the patient).

The difference between hearing and listening

Imagine lying in your bed in darkness and you are trying to sleep. Then you hear a noise at the window. (To hear is to become conscious of sound - without analysis). This hearing is followed by wondering, what is the cause of that sound? A burglar? A branch hitting the window? A son or daughter locked out? Now you are attentive to further sounds you are now listening. All of your being and will bends to understand, (detective like) to grasp the meaning or import of the sound.

For the physician, listening is also this leaning toward and reverence to the history. Listening is a patient-focused new-brain weighted activity. Hearing, by contrast, is a reptilian weighted activity, cocking an ear to self-interest, not the patient's.

We can, however, command the ability to listen. I have seen a physi-

LISTENING

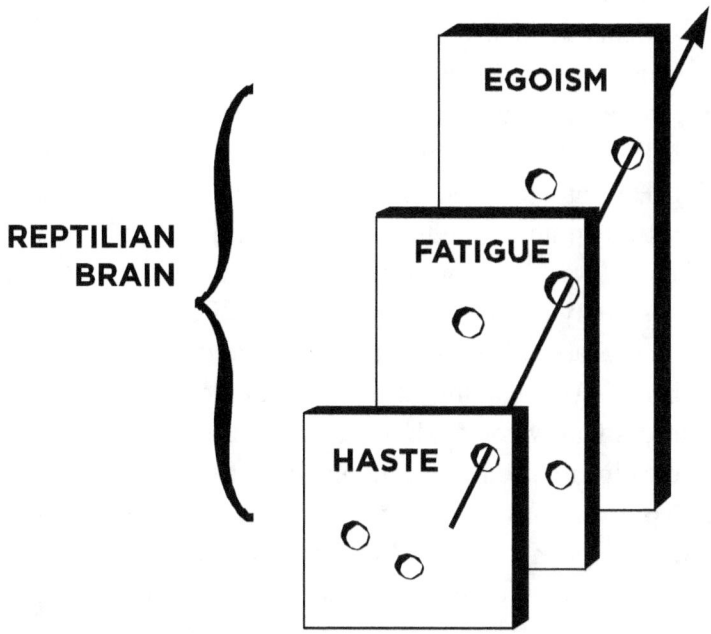

Figure 14 Barriers to Listening

cian listen to one patient with influence and talk-over another patient from a lower socio-economic group with similar symptoms. Notice the attention we can command to our mechanic, financial advisor or contractor? Notice also how easy it is to listen to praise or thanks (reptilian delectable data) and how difficult (how irritating) it is listen to challenges and criticisms (reptilian offensive data).

Why is it so difficult to listen?

We speak approximately 125-160 words a minute but we have the capacity to listen to 400 words per minute.[161] These gaps in listening can reflexedly be filled by our reptilian agenda of self-interests, assumptions, convenience and preservation of our hypothesis. The obstacles to listening are the same as those to good performance, listed in Chapter 6. The Inverted Swiss Cheese Model can also apply to good listening. (Figure 14)

The more one listens the more one learns about the patient.
Some patients are reluctant to give their symptoms. I recall an 82-year-old woman who presented to our emergency department at 1AM with a sore throat. She was triaged to the non-acute section of the department and waited three hours before I saw her. She had no trouble swallowing. Her throat looked normal and her vital signs were also normal. I sat down and talked about her life, her hobbies and her friends. Then as I was about to leave she says, "By the way doctor, I get this heaviness in my chest and it's worse when I do the housework. My doctor knows about it, I don't know why I told you – you seemed interested in me." After battling fatigue for a few hours, I wanted to say to her, "see your family doctor about it." Her E.C.G. showed ischemic changes, indicating reduced blood supply to the heart muscle.

Hints from doctors who didn't want to give their patients' tongues much airtime. Or further signs of burnout.

- One physician would stick a thermometer into the patient's mouth, when he did not wish the patient to talk.
- Another physician I knew had the front legs of the patients' bare wooden chair four inches shorter than the hind legs to discourage relating of history.[162] This practice contrasts with a doctor who used to offer his patients a glass of sherry to settle them.
- Another physician would drop the phone and complain about the bad connection.
- I knew another who'd lift his spectacles onto his forehead and allow the patient to talk till the spectacles dropped onto his nose, thus lowering the boom on the consultation.

What are the signs that we are not listening?
There are the generic signs and signs specific to listening which can warn us when we are not listening. The generic signs stem from reptilian attachment.

- Labeling, criticizing the patient, their relatives, their grammar, the staff, and the institution in which we work.

- Heightened irritability level is on our Irritability Barometer. The Pilot's Crew Resource Management Manual [163] lists other signs of inattention or distraction specific to listening. These signs depict more self-interest than patient interest.

- We pre-plan or formulate a response and do not listen to what the person is saying.

- We can detour. Lay in ambush for a key word, and when it comes up, we take the conversation into another area of our interest. We sometimes wait to snare the symptoms which are the least inconvenient for us.

- We debate: we play the devil's advocate, so that regardless of what is said, we might take the opposite point of view. I played the devil's advocate with the relatives and the attending nurse of the patient who had the volvulus. (Asserting one's intellectual territory).

- We interrupt frequently.

- We talk over, raise our volume and/or sharpen our tone.

Again, many of these signs resonate with Bergson's claim, *"we do not aim at knowledge for the sake of knowledge but in order to take sides, to draw profits, in short to satisfy our self-interest."*

But how can we become better listeners?
We live in a culture that discourages listening. For example, we practice not listening when the radio or T.V. drones in the background. The aviation industry prefers the term active listening to listening. Active listening depends on the presence of will, on leaning toward the patient's history, on vigilance to the task at hand. To improve our listening we need practice focusing on different aspects of listening.

Callisthenics for active listening
- Practice paying attention to listening especially listening to those you dislike or who challenge you. The more you practice being present to the other's voice, the easier you will be able to listen to the patient's.

- Have the radio or the T.V. on, only when you are able to give your full attention.

- Count how often you interrupt others when they talk. I found that to let the patient speak for three to five minutes without interruption seemed like an eternity.

- Observe if you finish the other's sentence.

- Listen to the quality of your verbal questions. Are they closed, open or probing? Do you ask the patient to elaborate?

- Do you paraphrase what the patient has said to ensure that you have understood the patient?

- Observe the quality of your non-verbal questions. Do you face the speaker? Are you relaxed? Do you make eye contact? Do you encourage the other to speak? Do you give patients the chance to tell their story?

- Do you talk over the other?

- Do you pre-plan?

- Do you debate?

- Do you lie in ambush?

- Are you critical of patients, their grammar, habits, etc.?

- Are you now more irritable?

Make a list of these exercises and practice one of them with every sixth patient. By practice and increasing the frequency of them, they can become a habit, a habit of self-reflection on how well one is actively listening. These callisthenics could easily be replaced if one cares and leans toward the history.[164]

Active listening is demanding. It requires discipline especially when we are stressed or when we are hearing conflicting data which requires us to un-name, to acknowledge the whisper of doubt within and, horrors of horrors, to circle back again to where we began.

CHAPTER 12

Listening for the Whisper of Doubt Within.

*"Sydenham was called 'a man of many doubts' and therein
lay the secret of his great strength." -Osler*

Many dismiss the value of doubting as dithering or unmanly. Yet the "manly" aviation industry values any expression of doubting. In its Crew Resource Management Manual, in large bold font, is the following directive: **"IF SOMETHING DOESN'T LOOK OR FEEL RIGHT, IT PROBABLY ISN'T."**

Doubt is often the only stop sign on the road to error. We can experience doubt weakly or strongly. For example, the KLM captain of the tragic flight 4805 at Tenerife doubted weakly, "… this caused some concern with KLM flight engineer asking the captain; 'is he not clear then?' After repeating his question, the captain answers emphatically, 'Oh, yes.'"

It is worth deliberating on the captain's emphasis. Why did the captain answer emphatically, rather than calmly? Emphatic expression is a spittle, spraying one's intellectual territory, discouraging further intrusion. And in that KLM cockpit, it discouraged further questioning.

There is another reason to be suspicious of emphatic expression. Newman claimed that "to say that something must be, is to admit that it may not be." A corollary of Newman's statement is also true, "to say that something must not be, is to admit that it might be." Likewise, Nobel Laureate, Medawar warned against emphatic expression, "The intensity of the conviction has no bearing on its veracity."[165]

Emphasis is a reptilian expression which paradoxically implies more doubt than certainty. Emphatic expression is not a prerequisite for clear communication. In the currency of communication, emphasis is an opaque shard of vigor and uncertainty which is often mistaken for a gem of clarity.

By contrast to the meekness of the KLM pilot's doubt, Dr. Chisholm's doubt scorched. *"I wake up at two o'clock in the morning in a sweat. 'Dead gut.' 'I missed dead gut.' Or maybe worse. And maybe worse it was necrotizing fasciitis. And I gave her enoxaparin… the surgeon will love that when he goes to the operating room. I toss and turn for another two hours before going back to sleep."*[166] I also awoke harboring certain doubt regarding my patient with the volvulus.

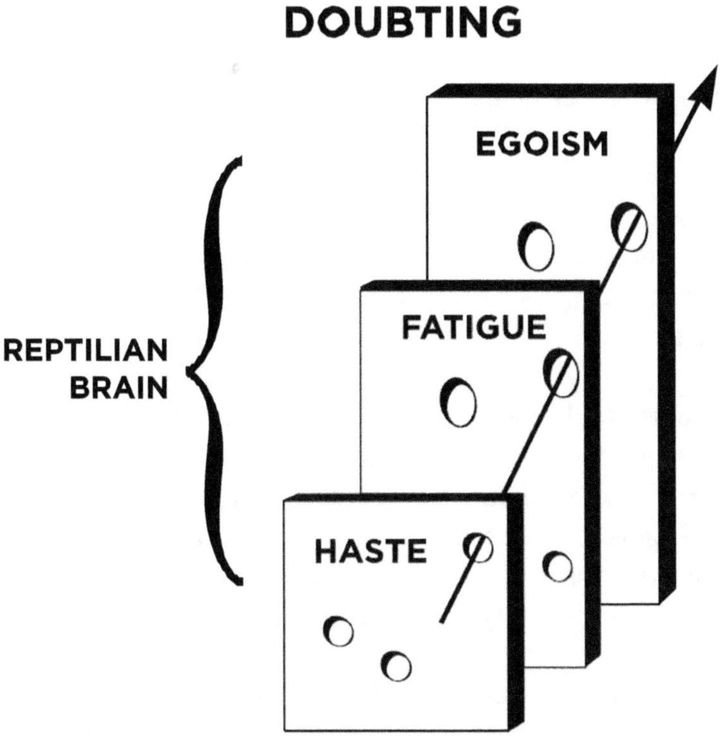

DOUBTING

Figure 15 Barriers to Doubting

When we sleep, we are detached from our reptilian influences, and upon wakening, we are unencumbered by our reptilian brain and can then doubt strongly, clearly and decisively, as Chisholm had.[167] The KLM captain, on the other hand, could not detach himself from his attachment to fly to Amsterdam that evening.[168]

The intensity of our doubting is inversely proportional to the intensity of **our attachments** to our reptilian influences. This relationship of doubt appreciation to reptilian attachment can be loosely depicted both by the following relationship and also by the Inverted Swiss Cheese Model (figure 15).

$$\text{Appreciating and receiving doubt} \propto \frac{1}{\text{Attachment to Reptilian Influence}}$$

Classification of doubt

Simone Weil, celebrated philosopher, claimed that, "Attachment is the great fabricator of illusions. Only those who are detached can appreciate reality."[169] Since doubt is often a necessary earlier process to reaching reality, what holds for appreciating reality also holds for appreciating doubt. We, therefore, can say only those who are detached can appreciate doubt. Doubt can be classified[170] into those detached from and those attached to our reptilian influences.

Detached doubt involves a carefree, discretionary activity, for example, sitting in the "lazy boy" and musing on a bridge, chess, or crossword puzzle. These activities do not prod our reptilian interests, such as haste and egoism; consequently, we experience little or no physical symptoms with this kind of doubting. Even with such cozy doubts, we often find that we solve these problems by walking away and returning later to them with "fresh, rested" eyes.

Attached doubts are those attached to our reptilian agendas, namely, self-esteem, haste and convenience. Attached doubts are inconvenient and uncomfortable because they reveal our uncertainty, humility and forecast more work. There are two types of attached doubts.

The unavoidable attached doubt is compelling. One can't avoid it because it challenges our self-interests, for example, losing one's way in a city and rushing to catch a plane. It shouts. One can't ignore or deny this doubt. It is our ignorance manifest. One is obliged to ask for help.

Dispensable attached doubt may not be as compelling as the unavoidable one. It often whispers and may be fleeting or niggling (recurring). Why one doubt niggles and another is fleeting can be as much dependent on the strength of our attachment to our reptilian influences as on the seriousness of the content of the doubt.

The pilot must be vigilant to both niggling and fleeting doubts, because his or her life is at stake. The difference between physicians' and pilots' valences to their work and doubting can be like the different valences the chicken and the pig bring to the breakfast. The chicken is involved but the pig is committed.[171]

Introduction to recognizing doubt's expressions

It is easy to recognize doubt when we are prompted by the questioning look or challenge of a patient, relative or nurse. Doubting, however, should not depend on their gumption to question us. The master attitude is to self-initiate doubt like Dr. Manson did in Cronin's vignette. Bergson claimed that intelligence is the power to ask questions of one's self, to initiate doubt. Doubting, however, is difficult because it challenges our self-esteem and also because it begs more effort and more of our time.

Toward effective self-questioning

Since doubting is difficult, how then do we become more open to our doubts? There are four steps.

- Learn and list the many expressions of our doubting.
- Test how receptive we are to doubt. Do we have the space within our agendas to doubt? If we don't, then…
- Find the space to doubt and finally …
- Pursue the lines of inquiry which doubt reveals.

Step One: Identifying the signs of doubting

The CRM Manual states "that the most detectable and reliable clue to the loss of Situational Awareness is gut feeling.[172] Our bodies are able to detect stimuli long before we have put the big picture together. Learn to recognize your own signs, such as stomach butterflies, muscle tension, mood swings, etc. Trust your feeling; policemen sometimes place their lives on their gut feelings."[173]

Subtle Signs of Doubting

It is easier to recognize the signs of doubt when they cause stomach butterflies (fear), muscle tension (anxiety), or mood swings (impatience) or when they are voiced by a colleague. But doubt may whisper only once, ectopic, sub-arachnoid, glaucoma. Doubt may not be as di-

101

rect as whispering a name. It may be:

- a snag in our verbal flow, such as a hesitancy in a few words, like the first officer from the cockpit voice recorder shows prior to the tragic accident in Cali, Columbia.

First Officer: "Uh, where are we… we going out to…"
Captain: "Let's right to, uh, Tulua first of all. OK?"
A few seconds later, Captain identifies Tulua.

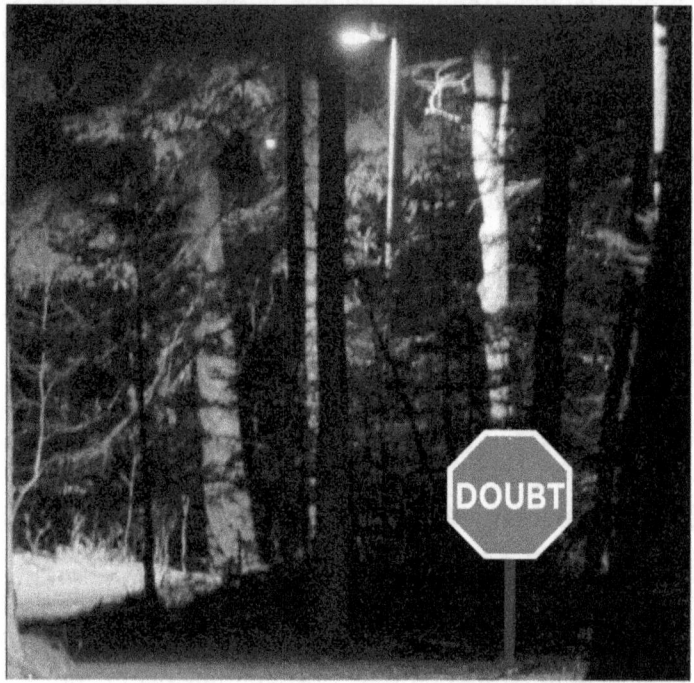

Figure 16 Doubt may the only stop sign on the road to error.

Captain: "Just doesn't look right on mine. I don't know why."
Two minutes later they impacted into a mountain.

- a less affirmative tone or a questioning inflection in the voice to what began as a statement
- an incompleted sentence
- difficulty to find an appropriate word to express a banal thought
- an emphasis in speech or posture

These discrete signs often appear at the conclusion of the consultation with the patient, when writing prescription or discharge instructions. Watch for them.

These signs are easier to see in others than in ourselves and more difficult to appreciate amid the exigencies of our practices. Remember doubt may be the only advocate for the patient's interest and the last stop sign on the path to error.

Step Two: Determining how receptive we are to doubt

- Before we begin a consultation we can ask ourselves do we have space for doubt, to initiate doubt and pursue its lines of inquiry? We can also ask the same questions toward the end of the consultation.

- Do we have the gumption to ask: "What else could this be?"

- How do we receive conflicting data, calmly, grudgingly, or with a hasty emphatic dismissal?

- We can also test our receptivity to conflicting data by imagining its arrival.

- We can ask ourselves if we like to be tended by a physician who might ignore doubt as we are contemplating now.

- Do we have the reserves to do the inconvenient, to un-name, to pursue other possibilities, to go "backwards?"

- How attached are we to the major reptilian influences, namely, haste, egoism, and apathy?

- One further test of confidence is to ask oneself: "Would I like to be treated as I am treating this patient?" To answer no, is a vote for reasonable doubt, for reassessment.

Step Three: Freeing space to doubt

Kierkegaard warned that we must keep our mind free from certainty like a port free from ice where we spent the winter. How can we thaw our minds, for conflicting data to surface and for doubt to navigate? To free space to doubt, we need to discover if haste, egoism and/or apathy is filling the space:

- To rule out haste, ask yourself whether you would explore the history more or treat differently if you had more time, or if the time of consultation was convenient for you; or whether you would consider and pursue the other possibility if you had thought of it at first.

- To rule out egoism, ask yourself whether your course of action

Haste	"Not so fast. Think first."
Egoism	It's not who is right, but what's right. The patient's well-being is more important than my self-esteem.
Tiredness - Apathy "What's the use?"	"I am not helpless, I can make a difference."
Convenience	Has little to do with quality work.
Labeling	Has little to do with pathology. Be aware of the distinction between concepts and reality. Here, the label is the concept.

Table 4 Specific Antidotes

would change if a different consultant was on call, or if the time of the referral was more convenient for the consultant; for example, if the consultant was present in the department.

- To rule out apathy, ask yourself whether your actions would change if this was a person dear to you or of influence.[174] Note how we improve our driving when a police car is behind us.

Antidotes

Should an obstacle be present, then employ the specific antidotes and generic antidotes as required. One may develop their own antidotes. Below I offer antidotes gleaned from various sources including the aviation industry. For specific antidotes see Table 4 below. Generic antidotes follow.

Reptilian Attitudes	Antidotes

Generic antidotes

- I have the freedom to do thorough work. Frankl: "It is not the situation but how we respond to it that defines us."

- Effort and inconvenience are often required for clarity. (After Bergson).

- Transpose oneself three months into the future. How small then becomes our present reptilian attachments from that distance? Or our reptilian attachments of three months ago are of little importance now. (Like Frankl discovered).

- Transpose the inconvenience of the moment to another physician's inconvenience. It would then ruffle our feathers less. (Epictetus recommended this transposition of problems).

- Sun Tsu observed, "anger with time can revert to joy." Similarly, irritability can revert to patience. Why not be patient now, when it matters?

Step Four: Pursuing the lines of investigations of doubt

Thomas Addison (1815-1860) provides an example of pursuing doubt. "He has also been known, after seeing a patient within the radius of eight or ten miles, to remember on his near approach to London, thinking over the case on his way, that he had omitted some seemingly important inquiry, and to have posted back some miles for the purpose of satisfying his mind on the doubt which had occurred to it."[175]

After acknowledging doubt, we should pursue new options. Talk to the patient again. Tease out the precise sequence of events. Contact relatives to clarify the history and determine why they were worried about their relative, what has changed? Examine more thoroughly an organ or system. Order a test. The pursuing of other options often may not be too demanding or time consuming, though neither of these should be a consideration in thorough work.

Callisthenics for appreciating doubt

- We can observe how differently we feel between detached doubt and attached doubt, for example, between solving a chess or bridge problem at home or in a tournament, or between hitting a golf ball on the practice range and on the first tee of a tournament.

- Observe how golfers or bridge players will hesitate or slow down in their speech when they doubt.

- Observe how we become distracted from the task at hand when we begin to doubt.

- Familiarize oneself with the physical sensations such as when you are lost in a city, forest or when asking a stranger for directions.

- Learn a foreign language or a new instrument. These are unending sources of doubt with their accompanying sentinel physical signs.

- Look for hesitancy when concluding the consultation or writing a prescription.

- Observe for any form of emphasis at home and at work. When one is emphatic one is more likely to be doubting and also more likely to dismiss doubt without flinching.

- Practice observing hesitancy in speech in ourselves, our patients and co-workers.

- Observe one's reaction to the patient's history. Are we more partial to one part than another? Partiality is a reptilian response that favors data that conforms to our hypothesis or convenience.

Callisthenics to initiate doubt

Regularly challenge ourselves.

- What else could this be?
- What else could have caused this?
- What else could complicate this?
- Did I order the right dosage for a patient?
- Did I check if that patient was allergic to that drug?
- Could there be a possible interaction among the patient's medications?

Make a list of these exercises and practice one of them with every sixth patient. By practice they can become a habit, a habit of self-reflection on how well we can appreciate and initiate doubt, and how willing we are to pursue its questions.

Further musings on doubt

It is easier to doubt in a field outside of one's specialty but it takes gumption to doubt in one's domain. We can also doubt our technical competence, for example, to intubate, to access a central line, to perform an ultrasound, perform a thoracenthesis, etc.

In Summary:

A Chinese Proverb says, to be uncertain is inconvenient, but to be certain is to be ridiculous. Regrettably, we are hard-wired to ignore doubt or to dismiss it without flinching. Paradoxically, doubt more than certainty should be reassuring to us, because when we doubt, we are more objectively involved with the puzzle. Pilots strive to appreciate any expressions of doubt. The physician should do the same.

Again there are four steps toward effective self-questioning mentioned earlier in the chapter.

We need to thaw the ice of certainty by imperturbability and by initiating the questions: What else could this be? What else could make this worse? Am I competent to do this? Would I like to be treated with the same doubts as I harbor now?

Whenever we see doubt we tend to shun her like a creditor. But shouldn't we search for doubt at the dance, ask her out and get to know her? Doubt is a true friend. Only a true friend will tell you that you've got dirt on your face.

INTRODUCTION TO PART V

"Know the Enemy"-Sun Tzu

The best physicians, like the best generals, are the ones who make the least mistakes.[176] Sun Tzu, in the Art of War, identified salient obstructions to good judgment: *"The flawed general is incapable of fathoming the enemy... easily angered, hasty to act and arrogant. "* Sun Tzu valued knowing the enemy.

"Know the enemy,
Know yourself,
And victory is never in doubt,
Not in a hundred years. "[177]

Sun Tzu also warned that, *"If you take your enemy lightly, he is likely to capture you. "*

Sun Tzu, to underscore the value of knowing the enemy, advises to *"Pay our spies well,..."* (because) *"... all strategies and techniques no matter how clear and varied cannot ensure victory without devoting a corresponding effort to fathoming and assessing the enemy. "*

Military strategists know that the enemy gets to vote on the outcome. The reptilian brain, the physician's enemy, also gets to vote on the outcome. It behooves us then to learn as much as we can about our enemy, our reptilian brain, which is as tireless as gravity. This concluding part has three chapters:

The first suggests callisthenics to train our attention and observing reptilian attachments. The second is a check list of our fitness to work. The final chapter provides an algorithm (The NewMind Response™) to employ from moment to moment at work.

PART V: THE NEWMIND RESPONSE™

CHAPTER 13

Callisthenics to improve recognition of reptilian attachment and vigilance to the task at hand.

Often those around us do not feel empowered to criticize our disposition or process. Even should that level playing field arrive, we should not rely on others to monitor our reptilian attachment. To im- prove our recognition of our reptilian attachment we can take one callisthenic and practice it all day long. Also, employ the specific antidote and/or generic ones. The next day, focus on another callisthenic. This process takes practice and gritty resolve, but we can improve our aware- ness of the reptile within. Changing a habit or poise is like climbing The Leaning Tower of Pisa.[178] At times we feel like we are descending and going in circles, but with perseverance we can make progress.

Daily Callisthenics

1. A day of monitoring our irritability levels by employing our Irritability Barometer, see Chapter 4. (Will not the musician tune the lute when it is out of tune? Epictetus).

2. A day of monitoring our interruptions of patients. Remind ourselves that the more we listen, the more we learn. Can we listen for three minutes without an interruption? We should observe for signs of our inattention and practice the callisthenics for active listening as out-

111

lined in Chapter 11.

3. A day of spotting our labeling of staff, patients, their relatives. Remind ourselves that labeling tempts different levels of care. Labeling reflects more our attachment to the reptilian influence than the patient's pathology.

4. A day without time pieces. To check the pulse and respiratory rates use a minute sand glass. In eight hours there are 480 minutes. These deliberate simple tasks are also opportunities to reflect on one's poise and reserve to do thorough work.

5. A day of noting the seduction of convenient ways. (Note the convenient might be the way we are most adept at performing a procedure. I mean by the word convenient, lazy. See No. 5 of the verbatim account from Chapter 1 for a clear example). The convenience antidote is effort, and effort is the clarity, the truth we seek.

6. A day of observing how attached we are to our self-image. Do we look at the on-call-list before we decide whether to call a consultant? Do we advocate differently depending on the consultant involved? How ready are we to accept challenging questions? Remember, we are paid to tend the patient not our self-image. Review Chapter 8.

7. A day of reviewing our ability to appreciate the whispers of doubt. See Chapter 12. Again, here are the four steps toward effective self-questioning.
- Learn and list the many expressions of our doubting.
- Test how receptive we are to doubt. Do we have the space within our agendas to doubt? If we don't, then…
- Find the space to doubt and finally…
- Pursue the lines of inquiry which doubt reveals.

8. A day of transposing ourselves three months into the future when we encounter doubt. Review Viktor Frankl's reflections in the section, "A Distant View of Climbing the Devil's Ladder toward the

Diagnosis", in Chapter 10.

9. A day of being able, when we are concluding the consultation, to have the reserve to ask the vital questions about each patient:
  - What else could this be?
  - Is this a symptom or a diagnosis?
  - What else could make this worse?
  - Would I like to be tended as I am tending now?

10. A day of appreciating the vital signs. Especially verify the respiratory rate and observe its characteristics. This sign is the one most likely to be inaccurate. The contemplation upon the vital signs is also an opportunity to reflect on our command or lack of imperturbability at that moment.

11. A day of categorizing our conclusions, like Osler instructs, *"Begin early to make a threefold category: clear cases, doubtful cases, mistakes. And play the game fair, no self–deception, no shrinking from the truth; mercy and consideration for the other man, but none for yourself, upon whom you have to keep an incessant watch... ... It is only by getting your cases grouped in this way that you can make any real progress in your post-collegiate education; only in this way can you gain wisdom with experience."*[179]

12. Each day practice vigilance to the task at hand, as outlined in Chapter 4. It is difficult to be vigilant to the task at hand. I find this easier to do when one's self interest is involved, for example, walking in water with jellyfish. For two weeks each year, jellyfish invade the Northumberland Straits. At that time, I can wade to and fro to a sand bar and watch for jelly fish for thirty minutes without losing this focus. Such a focus we should and can bring to the patient's history and examination.

Since we are hard-wired to react with our reptilian brain, how can we remember to perform these counter-reptilian callisthenics? Place a label on our clipboard, stethoscope or pen as a reminder. We can keep a score board of these activities. See how often we recall to do each item. The ones we most frequently forget to perform are the ones we need to practice more.

CHAPTER 14

The Physician Prepares for Work

"Every battle is won before it is fought." -Sun Tzu

We can monitor:
Burnout score every three months;
"Am I Safer" fitness to work daily;
And our poise throughout our day at work (Chapter 15)..

Every three months we can review ourselves for signs of burnout as out-lined in Chapter 9 and by using the same questionnaire and tracking our progress numerically.

Daily pilots inspect their fitness to fly by using the mnemonic "I'm safe." I add the letter R to this list for "rushed", making it "I'm safer". We physicians should also examine ourselves at the beginning of each shift or day at the office to gauge our space to do the inconvenient (Table 5).

These enhancers make it more difficult for us to appreciate the whispers of doubt, the spurs of haste, the hisses of irritability, the tasteless poison of sleep deprivation, the temptation of meritocracy when labeling, the seduction of the convenient and the treachery of egoism. These enhancers thereby lessen our objectivity and deplete our psychic energy to do the inconvenient, thorough work.

Identify and redress the reptilian brain enhancers outside and at work in the following table.

A doctor prepares to meet the day's work

I'	Illness	Am I feeling unwell?
M	Medication	Have I been taking any prescription, over- the- counter drugs, or illicit drugs?
S	Stress	Am I under acute or chronic psychological pressure from job, money, health or family?
A	Alcohol	Have I been drinking within the last eight hours?
F	Fatigue	Am I tired or sleep deprived?
E	Eating	Am I adequately nourished?
R	Rushed	Overbooked? Director requests more productivity from me? Delay in O.R.? Is the time of the consultation convenient for me?

Table 5 "Am I Safer?"

CHAPTER 15

THE NewMind RESPONSE™

Though we may have answered NO to the presence of reptilian brain enhancers, the reptilian brain persists in advocating its self interest which is at cross purposes to the patient's well-being. Therefore, it still needs monitoring. How can we monitor our attachment to reptilian demands? Future researchers might develop subtle instruments such as voice print, sweat gland activity, pupil size, blink rate or rhythm, respiratory rate or rhythm, pulse rate or rhythm, fasciculations of paravertebral muscles, or rhythms and patterns of hand movements. Some of these might correlate from moment to moment with levels of heightened reptilian attachments. I propose an algorithm (Figure 17, below) that hopefully in the future will prove rudimentary.

Algorithm for Heightened Reptilian Attachment
(Striving toward the NewMind Response™)

The algorithm (Figure 17) has three steps for monitoring, identifying and neutralizing heightened reptilian attachment.
Step 1. To identify heightened reptilian attachment, we ask ourselves five questions.
Step 2. If heightened reptilian attachment is present, we can identify its cause(s) by asking ourselves four questions.
Step 3. We employ appropriate antidote(s) (see specific antidotes, Table 3) together with or without generic antidotes (Chapter 12 and below) to counter heightened reptilian attachment.

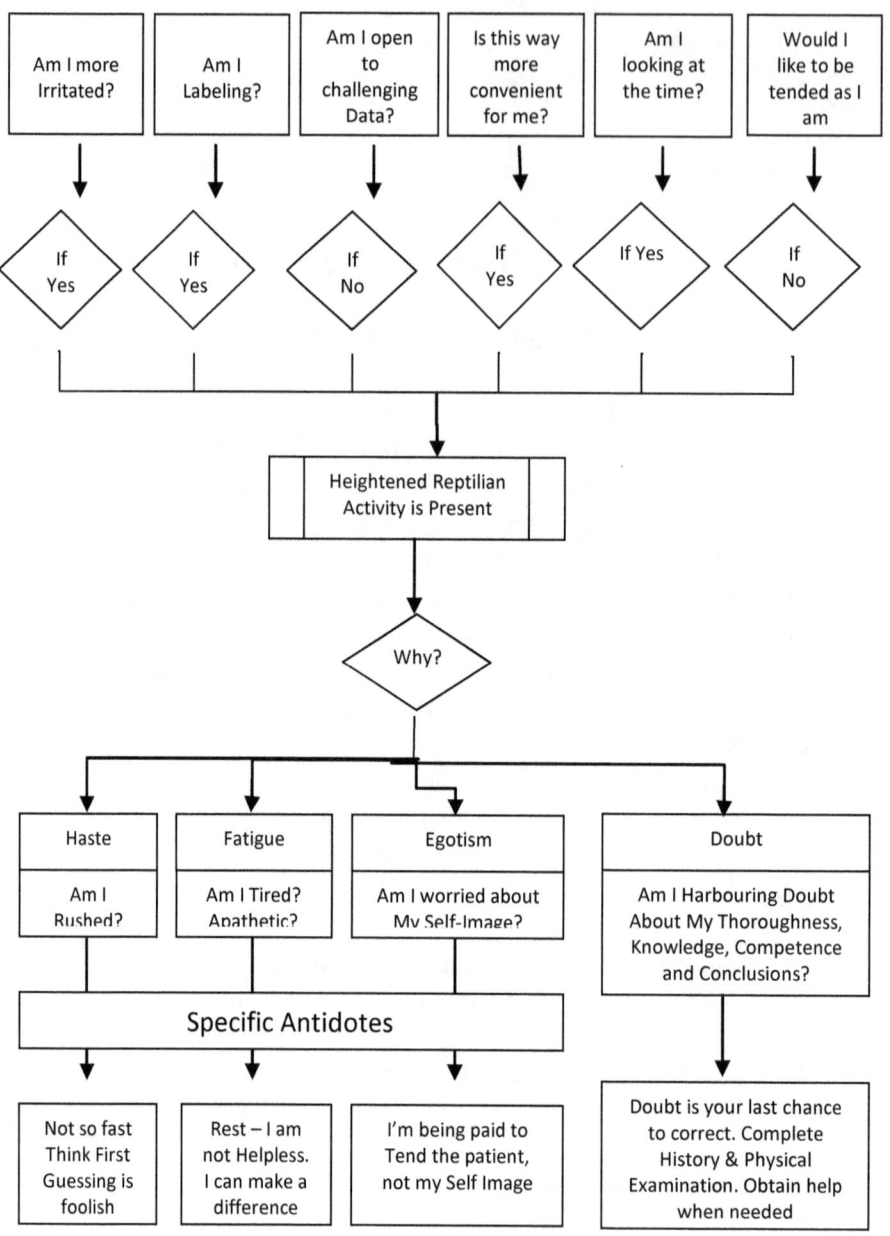

Figure 17 – Algorithm towards self-knowledge or towards heightened attachment to the reptilian brain.

Specific antidotes are listed in the **right column** below.

Haste	"Not so fast. Think first."
Egoism	It's not who is right, but what's right. The patient's well-being is more important than my self-esteem.
Tired, apathetic, "What's the use?"	"I am not helpless, I can make a difference."
Labeling	Will impede more than help diagnosing the patient.
Convenience	Effort is the clarity we seek.[i] The correct action is often the inconvenient. Stellar action is always inconvenient.

Generic antidotes are again listed here:

I have the freedom to do thorough work. Frankl: "It is not the situation but how we respond to it that defines us."
Effort and inconvenience are often required for clarity. (After Bergson).
Transpose oneself three months into the future. How small then becomes our present reptilian attachments from that distance? Or our reptilian attachments of three months ago are of little importance now. (Like Frankl discovered).
Transpose the inconvenience of the moment to another physician's inconvenience. It would then ruffle our feathers less.

(Epictetus recommended this transposition of problems).
Sun Tsu observed, "anger with time can revert to joy." Similarly, irritability can revert to patience. Why not be patient now, when it matters?

In Conclusion

The hypothesis is that error is an expression of our reptilian brain. We physicians should learn when our attachment to the reptilian brain is influencing our work. At the end of the consultation, we should command energy and clear a space within to answer truthfully the vital questions:

- What else could this be?
- Is this a symptom or a diagnosis?
- What else could make this worse?
- What is unique or different about this presentation?
- Whose interest is being served by this conclusion, the patient's or the physician's?
- In what way is the patient's condition different **now** than normally?
- Would I like to be tended as I am tending now?

Finally, what might patients expect from us? They might expect patience not irritability; genuine inquiry, not assumptions; attention to the task at hand, not day-dreaming; candor about our certain doubts, not duplicity about our doubtful certainties; and, when indicated, they might expect what is inconvenient for us, not what is convenient.

Throughout this book, I have neglected the patient, because by now we should realize that the patient we are working on is the patient called ourselves, whose symptoms are haste, egoism, and apathy and whose diagnosis is a space-occupying lesion, called the reptilian brain.[ii] While the lesion is inoperable and the prognosis for this condition is guarded, we can take hope that in a leaning tower, we can stand erect; that amid the profound depravities of labor camps, we can be altruistic; and that in the face of danger, we can command grace and humor. Surely then, amid the uncertainties, doubts, and demands of our medical practice, we can without any impatience reach after fact and reason.

The End[1]

_____

[1] The end is never reached because man still bears in his bodily frame the indelible stamp of his lowly origin.

APPENDIX 1

The incidence of medical errors

"Let them learn their art (medicine) properly or cease to practice it. A mistake in other professions is tolerable, but this is full of danger, if its practitioners are not perfect. It ravages like a hidden domestic plague." Marcellus Palingenius, physician, Venice 1500-43

Each generation rediscovers the truths of a previous one. Doctors rediscovered Palingenius' iatrogenic[183] hidden domestic plague about 450 years later when the Harvard Medical Practice Study I[184] and II[185] were published.[186]

Using weighed totals, the authors of the Harvard Study estimated that among the 2,671,863 patients discharged from New York State Hospitals in 1984, there were:

27,179 adverse events involving negligence.

6,895 deaths and 877 cases of permanent and total disability involving negligence in New York State in 1984.

Under the tort system, all of these could have led to successful litigation. The authors claimed, "Because our sample of hospital records was random, we could provide for the first time population estimates of adverse events and adverse events due to negligence."[187] As the authors extrapolated for the state of New York, I extrapolated these results to the U.S.A. In the Orwellian Year of 1984, in the U.S.A., there were about 82,740 deaths due to preventable medical error.

In the six months following this publication, there was not one letter to the editor of the New England Journal of Medicine on this study. It seemed that either doctors were overwhelmed by this report card or held their noses and hoped that the stench would somehow disappear. It didn't.

The findings of the Harvard Medical Practice Study in New York have been corroborated by a study of adverse events in Colorado and Utah occurring in 1992.[188] While the study in New York found that 13.6 percent of adverse events led to death, the Colorado and Utah study found that 6.6 percent of adverse events lead to death. This study implies that at least 44,000 Americans die in hospitals each year as a result of preventable medical errors.

Extrapolating these rates to the last twenty years in non-psychiatric American hospitals, one reaches the incredible conclusion that between 800,000 and 1,600,000 died from preventable medical errors.[189] Do not confuse the unbelievable with the untrue.

Some further reflections on the Harvard Medical Practice Study

Some maintain that these extrapolations likely underestimate the occurrence of preventable adverse events because these studies:

(1) considered those patients whose injuries resulted in a specified level of harm;

(2) imposed a high threshold to determine whether an adverse event was preventable or negligent (concurrence of two reviewers);[190]

(3) included only errors that were documented in patient records; and

(4) Hospital patients represent only a fraction of the total population at risk of experiencing adverse events such as, medications dispensed by pharmacies, patients treated as out-patients, patients in doctors' offices, in nursing homes, in ambulatory care clinics and those errors that did not result in injury.

Three further studies, respectively by Steel,[191] Andrews,[192] and Clarke,[193] which relied on both medical record abstraction and other information sources such as provider reports, have found higher rates of adverse events occurring in hospitals.

In the Steel study of 815 consecutive patients on a general medical service of a university hospital, it was found that 36 percent had an iatrogenic illness, defined as any illness that resulted from a diagnostic procedure, from any form of therapy, or from a harmful occurrence that was not a natural consequence of the patient's disease. Of the 815 patients, nine percent had an iatrogenic illness that threatened life or produced considerable disability, and for another two percent, iatrogenic illness was believed to contribute to the death of the patient.

In the Andrews study of 1047 patients admitted to two intensive care units and one surgical unit at a large teaching hospital, 480 (45.8 percent) were identified as having had an adverse event, where adverse event was defined as "situations in which an inappropriate decision was made when at the time, an appropriate alternative could have been chosen." For 185 patients (17.7 percent), the adverse event was serious, producing disability or death. The likelihood of experiencing an adverse event increased about six percent for each day of hospital stay. The likelihood of experiencing a serious adverse event increased about two percent for each day of hospital stay.

In the Clarke study of trauma resuscitation, reasoning errors were found in 100% of cases studied.

Wilson et al[194] reported that adverse events were associated with 17% of hospital admissions in Australia. Davies and colleagues[195] reported 21% of 4,000 charts reviewed in New Zealand contained evidence of adverse events. In acute care Canadian hospitals, errors or adverse events were estimated to occur in 7.5% of patient admissions each year.[196]

Seven years after the Harvard Medical Practice Study, the Institute of Medicine established the Quality of Health Care in America Committee with the charge of developing a strategy that will result in a threshold improvement in quality over the next ten years. Within two years, it produced a report to "break this cycle of inaction. " In its report, called "To Err is Human," the committee writes,[197] "despite the cost pressures, liability constraints, resistance to change and other seemingly insurmountable barriers, it's simply not acceptable to be harmed by the same health care system that is supposed to offer healing and comfort.... Given current knowledge about the magnitude of the problem, the committee believes it would be irresponsible to expect anything less than a 50% reduction in errors over five years."[198]

APPENDIX 2

The Neglect of Error by Medical Schools

The most fruitful lesson is the conquest of one's own errors. Whoever refuses to admit error may be a great scholar but he is not a great learner. Whoever is ashamed of error will struggle against recognizing and admitting it, which means that he struggles against his greatest gain. Goethe, *Maxims and Reflections.*

The professors at my medical school did emphasize diligence to history taking and physical examination. Only once, however, during my medical school did I remember an account of a lethal mistake.[199] Dr. de Valera, a consultant gynecologist recounted: "Professor Healy was Master of Holles Street Hospital and one day a woman was referred to him from a country doctor. He examined her and gave her a letter to give to her doctor. When she alighted from the train at Thurles Railway Station, she collapsed dead on the platform. Professor Healy turned to me and said; 'Ectopic pregnancy was one thing that I thought I knew something about.'"

Our neglect of mistakes is reflected in our vocabulary. We have in- vented names for the study of almost everything else from phrenology to astrology, and we even have a name for the study of knowing, epistemology, but none for the study of not knowing. This oversight is a testament to our hubris that we have not invented a word for the study of errors.

To name the study of error, I propose the neologism hamartology[200] derived from the Greek. The meaning in Greek has evolved from "to miss the target" to mean "the tragic flaw." The first meaning is the effect, the second is an explanation for the miss.

By studying our mistakes we succeed for our greatest gain. Some Medical Schools are beginning to redress this neglect. Dalhousie Medical School has introduced such a course on critical thinking. Its leading proponent Dr. Croskerry claims: "Currently, in medical training, we fail to recognize the importance of critical thinking and critical reasoning. The implicit assumption in medicine is that we know how to think. But we don't."

APPENDIX 3

Professionalism

One of the best definitions of a professional is given by the U.S. Congress in the Labor Management Relations Act 1047. According to this Act, a professional employee is one

- *Who is engaged in predominantly intellectual work, and is varied, as opposed to routine mental, mechanical, physical work*

- *Who is involved in the exercise of discretion and judgment in his or her work*

- *Whose output produced or the result accomplished cannot be standardized in relation to a given period of time*

- *Requiring knowledge of an advanced type in a field of science or learning customarily acquired by a prolonged course of specialized intellectual study in an institution of higher learning, as distinguished from a general academic education or from an apprenticeship.*

In addition to these criteria, other requirements are often added:

- *Professional registration requirements*
- *Activity in a professional society and other professional activities*
- *Public service nature of the occupation*
- *Adherence to a professional code of conduct and ethics.*

The third point above is one which many medical directors forget. They believe that the output produced or the result accomplished can be standardized in relation to a given period of time.

The Crew Resource Management Manual for Pilots also addresses professionalism.

- "PROFESSIONALISM in all its manifestations involves the discipline in the exercise of discretion and judgment in his or her work. The aviation industry believes that professionalism is found in an attitude of safety.

- Safety is an attitude, a frame of mind. It is being aware of one's environment and actions at all times. It requires intelligence and a reasonable ability to see, listen, and think.

- Safety is not something you can take or leave alone. It is not an activity that you participate in only when being watched or supervised.

- Safety is not posters, slogans or rules, nor is it movies, meetings, investigations or inspections.

- Ignoring safety does not indicate bravery, only foolishness. Conducting business in a safe and correct manner is the mark of a wise person, not a timid person.

In the end, for the pilot it is attention to detail that makes the difference, that separates the safe from the careless, and sometimes the living from the dead."

Finally, professionalism is the attention we bring to our work when someone, who is both authorative and knowledgeable, is watching us work. Two examples have been described. The first is how our driving improves when we notice a police car behind us. The second is Dr. Manson's imagining the nurse he admired was now watching him at work. Professionalism is when, by the spur of self-monitoring, we are attentive to the process.

APPENDIX 4

Relationships to complement the Inverted Swiss Cheese Model

We are striving for New Brain activities: Attention to the task at hand, active listening, discernment, doubting and doing the inconvenient. Our ability to perform these activities is dependent on the strength of attachment we have to our reptilian brain. This process can also be expressed by the following similar relationships.

$$\text{The Patient's Well-being} \propto \frac{\text{Attachment to the New Brain}}{\text{Attachment to the Reptilian Brain}}$$

$$\text{Attention to the task at hand} \propto \frac{\text{Attachment to the New Brain}}{\text{Attachment to the Reptilian Brain}}$$

$$\text{Doing the Inconvenient} \propto \frac{\text{Attachment to the New Brain}}{\text{Attachment to the Reptilian Brain}}$$

$$\text{Discernment} \propto \frac{\text{Attachment to the New Brain}}{\text{Attachment to the Reptilian Brain}}$$

$$\text{Doubting} \propto \frac{\text{Attachment to the New Brain}}{\text{Attachment to the Reptilian Brain}}$$

APPENDIX 5

William Osler's Bed-side Library for Medical Students

Osler writes: "A liberal education may be had at a very slight cost of time and money. Though the day be filled with appointed tasks, to make the best possible use of your talents, rest not satisfied with this professional training, but try to get the education, if not of a scholar, at least of a gentleman. Before going to sleep read for half an hour, and in the morning have a book open on your dressing table. You will be surprised how much can be accomplished in the course of a year. I have put down a list of ten books which you may make close friends. There are many others; studied carefully in your student days these will help in the inner education of which I speak.

The Old and New Testament
Shakespeare
Montaigne
Plutarch's lives
Marcus Aurelius
Epictetus
Religio Medici
Don Quixote
Emerson
Oliver Wendell Holmes—Breakfast – Table Series.
I have found the following helpful:
Man's Search for Meaning, by Viktor Frankl
Osler's collected addresses under the title: Aequanimitas
The Discourses of Epictetus
Iron Doc, by Dr. Mamta Gautam
Zen and the Art of Motorcycle Maintenance, by Robert Pirsig

Professional Pilot's Crew Resource Management Manual, by The Moncton College.

The Miracle of Mindfulness, by Thich Nhat Hanh

Be Free Where You Are, by Thich Nhat Hanh

Hamlet on the problems of doubt, proof and subjectivity

The Art of War, by Sun Tzu

Bhagavad-Gita

Chan Tzu

Tao Te Ching

Process: Introducing Themselves to Young (Christian) Minders, by Philip McShane

A Guide to the Good Life, by William B. Irvine

The Death of Ivan Illych, by Leo Tolstoy

APPENDIX 6

A Map of the Links at Krewe Island Spring 1931

Many books on sports and business focus on self-reflection and vigilance to the task at hand. They echo Krishna advice to Arjuna before battle: " Look to the action and not the fruits of the action." A recent variation on the Bhagavad Gita is the Legend of Bagger Vance (subtitled A Novel of Golf and the Game of Life) by Steven Pressfield. The Map of the Links at Krewe Island Spring 1931 highlights the internal bunkers, roughs and fairways in the game of thinking.

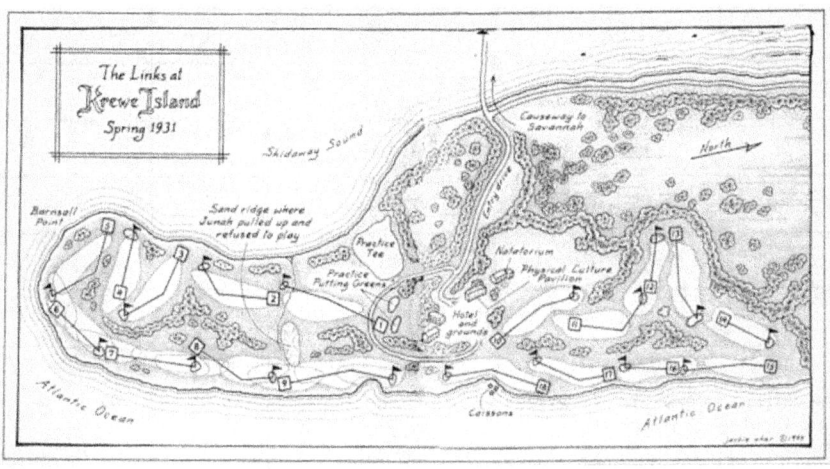

Names of the holes from 1 to 18:

Total 6854 Yards Par 72

Hole	Name	Championship Tees	Par	Handicap
1	Vigilance	521 yards	5	11
2	Sagacity	390 yards	4	13
3	Fortitude	325 yards	4	7
4	Prowess	194 yards	3	17
5	Rigor	378 yards	4	15
6	Temerity	230 yards	3	3
7	Cunning	405 yards	4	9
8	Might	442 yards	4	5
9	Faith	590 yards	5	1
10	Vigor	464 yards	4	6
11	Acumen	315 yards	4	14
12	Ingenuity	167 yards	3	8
13	Love	445 yards	4	18
14	Discipline	183 yards	3	10
15	Stamina	510 yards	5	16
16	Audacity	310 yards	4	12
17	Prudence	444 yards	4	4
18	Valor	541 yards	5	2

ACKNOWLEDGMENTS

For help in the long task of making this readable, I wish to thank Dr. Stephen Campbell of Grand Barachois, Mr. Bill Dekle of Claremore, and Dr. Brian Keogh of Grenoble. I also wish to thank Dr. Allison Dysart's Socratic examination, and subsequent directions which give this project a broader footing. Also thanks to Dr. Louis Crowe of Dublin for his generous counsel.

I am indebted to many more in various stages of this project: Mr. Robert Shaw for the illustrations and patience, and to Mr. Chris Tucker for cover design, which I chose for unalloyed reptilian baiting. To Mr. Bryan Copeland for guidance toward publishing this manuscript.

To Ms Jamie K. Morry for making this an Easter Sunday Morning Version. Many more for their enthusiasm and help: Dr M. Gautam M.O.T. for her generosity with Irondoc text, Dr. Arthur Armstrong, Dr. Kevin Black, Dr. Doug Mantz, Dr. David Symington, Dr. Michael Johnson, Mr. Ed Lamond, Ms. Elaine Amyot, Ms. Dawn Arnold, Dr. Mark Messenger, Mr. Lauchlin MacDowell, Dr. Ashwini Joshi, Dr. Gordon Dow, Ms. Louis Parent, Ms. Andrea Belliveau, Ms. Lise Godbout, Ms. Adeline Gibb, Ms. France Talbot, Mr. Eugene LeBlanc, Mr. Roy Gould, Mr. Gair Maxwell, Ms. Marilyn Macdonald, Dr. Andrew Boghen, Mr. Serge Morin, Dr. Andrew Clark, Mr. Martin Muldoon, my late father, Mr. James F. Meagher, Mr. Chris Morry, Dr. Philip McShane, Ms. Grace Morris, Jodie Brown-MacNamara R.N., Mr. Peter Gorman Jr., Dr. Al Fownes, Mr. Bill Hegan, Ms. Karen Fullerton B.Sc., Dr. Ron Garston, Dr, Joe Donachie, Dr. John Crompton, Dr. Gilbert

Quartey, Dr. Amal Bensaleh-Ratmi, Mr. Jean- Francois LeBlanc, Dr. Peter Jackson, Dr. James Crowley, Dr. Catherine Aquino Russell, Dr. Chris Losier, Dr. Gary Duguay, Dr. Serge Melanson, Dr. Luella Smith, Mr. Henrich Sirucek, Dr. R.M.M.S. Abeysekera, Mr. Tyler Hicks, Dr. Michael Greschener, Mr. Bill Bishop, Dr. Pat Croskerry, Dr. Paul Dubois, Mr. James Reason, Dr. Denise Dovovan, Dr. Brendan Kenny, Dr. Roderick Canning, Dr. Patrick O'Regan, Dr. Martin Shine, Dr. Marc Blayney, Dr. Gilles Cormier, Mr. Peter Sawyer, Ms. Susan Pickett, Ms. Lori Leger, Ms. Karen Darrach, Ms. Shannon MacTavish, Ms. Dorine Gagnon, Ms. Joyce Patriquin, The Staff of the Moncton Public Library, Mr. Jack Fritz, Mark Loeffler, and Don Loney; Mr. Mel Benson and Mr. Mike Doiron of the Moncton Flight College for allowing me to attend CRM lectures. To the Tatramar Seniors' College, especially Ms. Joan Beswick for her diligent reading and apt suggestions, and to the rest of the Focus Group, Ms. Judith Hubbard, Ms. Wallie Simieritsch and Mr. Tim Coates. Finally, I wish to thank Roisin for her enthusiasm, critique, support and efforts to have this published, to Cormac for his interest, Cashel for his suggestions, and Conor and Ruairi for their invaluable help with computers. To Bernie, for her poetry, art, Keatsian truth and for filling my journey with love for both me and our family.

REFERENCES AND NOTES

[1] "To Err is Human," Committee on Quality of Health Care in America; Institute of Medicine, National Academy Press Washington D.C.2001

[2] For further reflections on the incidence of medical errors see Appendix 1.

[3] Osler stressed the value of studying one's errors. "Start out with the conviction that absolute truth is hard to reach in matters relating to our fellow creatures, healthy or diseased, that slips in observation are inevitable even with the best trained faculties, that errors in judgment must occur in the practice of an art which consists largely in balancing probabilities; start, I say with this attitude of mind, and mistakes will be acknowledged and regretted; but instead of a slow process of self-deception, with ever-increasing inability, to recognize truth, you will draw from your errors the very lessons which may enable you to avoid their repetition." -Osler

[4] Increased Blood Urea Nitrogen (B.U.N.) usually is due to insufficient filtering of the blood by the kidney. In this case the insufficient filtering was due to depleted volume.

[5] The vital signs are heart and respiratory rates, blood pressure and temperature. The vital signs are vital, like stop signs. Like stop signs, sometimes if we ignore them, nothing happens, other times we crash.

[6] The term "sharp ends" is applied to describe "... the technical work of practitioners ....in the complex, rapidly changing, intrinsically hazardous world of health care." Cook RI, Render M, Woods DW. "Gaps in the continuity of care and progress on patient safety." British Medical Journal 2000; 320: 791-4.

[7] "Framing effect. How diagnosticians see things may be strongly influenced by the way in which the problem is framed." Croskerry P.

The Importance of Cognitive Errors in Diagnosis and Strategies to Minimize Them, Acad. Med. 2003; 78:775-780.

[8] Mediocrity is often dangerous, but never more dangerous than when it is given a euphemistic name.

[9] By not confessing I would hopefully avoid ridicule by my nurses and colleagues. I have seen doctors willing to criticize their peer's fall from grace. For example, one specialist queried if any of a colleague's fontanels had yet closed, and another avowed that he would not let an individual surgeon operate on any of his animals especially his retriever. By my silence, I might also dodge litigation and prevent the knowledge of my incompetence cascading down to the general public. A good name is easily lost: the quickest horse cannot overtake the spoken word. And when a good name is lost, it is lost forever. Could I, should I, ever practice again? My patients would constantly doubt me. I would have to leave town. "He, who steals my purse, steals trash. But he who steals my good name, steals all that I have." Iago in *Othello*.

[10] Christensen J F. *et al*. *The Heart of Darkness*. J Gen Intern Med. 1992; Vol 7 (July/August): 424-431. This article describes how physicians think and feel about perceived mistakes. A nurse friend, after being responsible for her patient's bad outcome, feeling unredeemable, considered throwing herself under a car shortly as she left the hospital.

[11] Shortly after, I saw the picture of a deer on the cover page of the National Geographic. I could see that its nostrils quivered for any strange scent, its eyes bulged for any egregious tremor of a limb and its ears pivoted for any snap or click of a twig, that the hunter might have overlooked. Isn't the diagnosis like a nervous flighty deer? One snap of a neglected symptom or sign and the diagnosis has bolted. Certainly, I had not stalked the diagnosis like the hunter its prey. I had lunged at it and it had slipped through my fingers.

There and then, I resolved never again to lunge at a diagnosis, but to stalk it. Lying on the table was a Canadian 10-dollar bill. It shows an osprey flying away with a fish in its talons. For hours, I have watched the ospreys fish near my cottage. They circle and circle slowly, then hover and go to dive only to swoop out of the dive and circle again and hover and dive and swoop yet again out of the dive. The ospreys might check themselves three times before their final buckle and hurl for the fish, which they nearly always bag. What causes the osprey to check its hurl, a shift of wind, a dysrhythmic wave, a change in the fish's tack?

There are different kinds of hunters. My cat will sit patiently for long times at the edge of the long grass, not distracted but focused, by the task at paw. He will often catch a mouse. My dog, like myself, is easily distracted. (There are numerous distractions to the doctor's work). My dog will turn from a pointed pheasant, to snap at a fly. The pheasant dashes off. Then there are the scavengers, who catch up with their kill when its prey is dead. I've done this too. We have the choice to be the imperturbable cat, the obsessive osprey, the easily distracted dog or the dead sure scavenger.

[12] Reason, James; Human Error, New York: Cambridge University Press. 1990

[13] Perceived Causes of Family Physicians' Errors, John W. Ely, MD. MSPH; Wendy Levison, MD; Nancy C.Elder, MD, MSHP; Arch G. Mainous111, Ph.D and Daniel C.Vinson, MD, MHSP. The Journal of Family Practice, Vol. 40, No.4(Apr), 1995

[14] Christensen J F. et al. see above. In contrast to the Ely group, these accounts were recorded in the third person.

[15] By convenience, I mean the lazy, slacker's way. Indeed, the convenient technique may be the way one is most adept in performing a procedure, but by convenience, I mean the lazy way. It will be a recurring theme that good work is often inconvenient and stellar work is always inconvenient. This last observation I heard from Dr.Gordon Dow.

[16] A Professional Pilot's Crew Resource Management Manual, volume I, page 1. Copyright Moncton Flight College. Crew Resource Management (CRM) training originated from a NASA workshop in 1979 that focused on improving air safety. The NASA research presented at this meeting found that the primary cause of the majority of aviation accidents was human error, and that the main problems were failures of interpersonal communication, leadership and decision making in the cockpit. A variety of CRM models have been successfully adapted to different types of industries and organizations, all based on the same basic concepts and principles. It has recently been adopted by the fire service to help improve situational awareness on the fire-ground.

[17] Crew Resource Management Manual, Copyright @ Moncton

Flight College.

[18] Haste, Egoism and Apathy could be called "The Terrible Three's."

[19] The limbic system is embryologically older than the new brain. It developed to manage 'fight' or 'flight' chemicals and is an evolutionary necessity for reptiles as well as humans. Recent studies of the limbic system of tetrapods have challenged some long-held tenets of forebrain evolution. The common ancestors of reptiles and mammals had a well-developed limbic system in which the basic subdivisions and connections of the amygdalar nuclei were established. Bruce LL, Neary TJ (1995)."The limbic system of tetrapods: a comparative analysis of cortical and amygdalar populations". Brain Behav. Evol. 46 (4–5): 224–34

[20] Frankl was interred for three years in Nazi death camps during The Second World War. This book was later published under the title, "Man's Search for Meaning", Washington Square Press Publications, New York, 1985. All quotations I attribute to Frankl are from this later title. I am indebted to Dr. Louis Crowe for recommending and giving me this book.

[21] Frankl V. E. "Man's Search for Meaning." Copyright © 1959, 1962, 1984, 1992 by Viktor E. Frankl. Reprinted by permission of Beacon Press, Boston.

[22] From a letter by Keats to his brothers, George and Tom, 1817.

[23] Chisholm C, Croskerry P.: A Case Study in Error: the Use of the Portfolio Entry. Academic Emergency Medicine 2004; 11: 388-392. Dr. Chisholm is to be commended for relating his thoughts and emotions so faithfully, as he managed a difficult patient in his emergency department. The authors "hoped that such candid discussions of errors in thought and action would reassure residents that the culture of "blame and shame," would not be part of their EM residency training, thereby encouraging error discussion and reporting. In addition, the fact that a senior-level faculty member candidly discussed these issues may reassure novices that they are not unusual and that protective strategies in clinical practice are a critical component of their lifelong learning."

[24] The journey, I suggest, might have been 1200 KM, from Florida to Indianapolis?

[25] Dr. Chisholm's encounter is also analyzed by Dr. Croskerry. To read, see Chisholm C, Croskerry P., cited above.

[26] Some people do not experience these awaking epiphanies.

[27] Kazantzakis Nikos, "Report to Greco," Simon and Schuster, New York 1965.

[28] Pirsig Robert, "Zen and the Art of Motorcycle Maintenance, an Inquiry into Values" Bantam Edition April 1975, New York, New York.

[29] Racker, a psychologist, called this detachment, an island of contemplation when he wrote of the need for rational faculty:

"There appears to be universal consensus that the patient can never be blamed for all the feelings experienced by the therapist."

"Adequate countertransference experience depends on.….The degree to which he (the analyst) is able, in his turn, to perform for himself what he so often performs for the patient, namely, to divide his ego into an irrational part that experiences and another rational part that observes the irrational part. Strive to find an island of contemplation from which the analyst can observe."

Transference and Countertransference by Heinrich Racker. International University Press Inc. New York 1968

[30] The summation of our attachments to the two brains can be also expressed as:

λ(Reptilian Brain Attachments) + (1-λ)(New Brain Attachments). (λ be $0 \leq \lambda \leq 1$).

[31] Bergson Henri, "Introduction to Metaphysics." G.P. Putman's Books, New York, 1912.

[32] The new-brain has developed rapidly while the reptilian brain has stalled by comparison. Julian Huxley observed: "cultural evolution proceeds at a rate hundreds of times that of biological evolution."

Consider the following timetable:

3,000,000 years ago: hominids bid goodbye to the apes

2,000,000 years ago: first tools created

150,000 years ago: first rock carvings and paintings

60,000 years ago: first flowers found in graves

45,000-35,000 years ago: modern man appeared; language evolved

40,000 years ago: first use of fire

13,000 years ago: grain was ground

10,000 years ago: last Ice Age ended

9,500 years ago: first complicated settlement

7,000 years ago: early switch from hunting and gathering to agriculture

5,500 years ago: the Old Kingdom of Egypt. (from "Emotional Common Sense" by Rolland S. Parker, Harper & Row, Publishers, Inc., New York, 1973)

For 50,000 human generations our basic neural circuitry was hard-wired for hunting and escape, whose reactions are fright, fight or flight, which do not accommodate to consideration, discernment and re-vision.

[33] Crew Resource Management Manual, Copyright, Moncton Flight College, NB., Canada

[34] From "Introduction to Metaphysics" by Henri Bergson

[35] From Dr. Gordon Dow in conversation.

[36] Even in a simpler time, attention was difficult. My uncle John, a priest, wondered how well his parishioners prayed. He stopped the horse he was riding by the side of a farmer. "See this horse here, four-year old gelding? Well broken in. I'll give it to you if you can say the Our Father without thinking of anything else but the words in the Our Father. Would you care to try? Just say it out loud when you are ready." The farmer wiped his brow, steadied himself by gripping the saddle, closed his eyes and began: "Our Father who art in heaven, hal- lowed be Thy name, Thy Kingdom come, Thy will be done on earth as it is in heaven. Will you throw in the bridle or saddle for luck?"

[37] Dehydration can be suspected, if one picks up the skin on the back of the hand and upon letting it drop it will remain elevated, that is tented, for a few seconds.

[38] Frankl maintained that we are defined more by our response to the system than the system in which we practice. Frankl questioned if some of the guards were less brutal than some of the prisoners. Just as we know the tree by its fruits, can we know the doctors by the accuracy and inaccuracy of their diagnoses? Through the autopsy of our errors, we learn that there is no cleavage between the diagnosis and the diagnostician, between conduct and character. I have found that error explored is a burst of meaning, of the unexpected, of a self-epiphany

into a world otherwise flattened out by non reflection.

[39] This phrase is taken from "The Object Stares Back: On The Nature of Seeing", by James Elkins, Harcourt Brace & Company, San Diego. 1997

[40] Diphthong is where two vowels are pronounced as one.

[41] Reason, James. "Human Error", New York: Cambridge Univer- sity Press, 1990

[42] Osler thought that of all men in the profession, the forty-visit a day man is the most to be pitied.

[43] Menachem Begin, the Israeli Prime Minister was a prisoner of the KGB in Russia. He described his experience of sleep deprivation as follows: "In the head of the interrogated prisoner, a haze begins to form. His spirit is wearied to death, his legs are unsteady, and he has one sole desire to sleep... Anyone who has experienced this desire knows that not hunger and thirst are comparable to it."

[44] Laurenson J. Sleep disturbance and performance. Anaesthesia, 2003, 58, pp. 1023-45.

[45] Barger Laura K, et al., Extended Work Shifts and the Risk of Motor Vehicle Crashes among Interns. N Engl J Med 2005; 352: 125-34

[46] Landrigan CP, et al. Effect of Reducing Interns' Work Hours on Serious Medical Errors in Intensive Care Units. N Engl J Med 2004; 351: 1838-48.

[47] Ely, et al. Perceived Causes of Family Physicians' Errors, see above

[48] Christensen J. F. et al, see above.

[49] Dawson, D. and Reid, K. Fatigue and alcohol intoxication have similar effects on performance. Nature, 1997; 388:235

[50] Fairclough, SH, Graham R, Impairment of Driving Performance Caused by Sleep Deprivation or Alcohol: A Comparative Study. Human Factors, Vol.41, No1 March 1999, pp. 118-128. A colleague of mine claims that there exists a bell curve distribution to the tolerance of sleep deprivation. He, for example, flew east two hours one day in a plane and worked the mid-night shift only to realise that he had to work the following day shift as well. He had a half hour nap between these two shifts. After that shift, he assisted a surgeon in the O.R. and then saw two patients in consultation in the emergency department. Following this, he drove to a poker game where he had eight beers and

151

won money! He drove home to sleep after being awake for over forty hours. He claims that there is a bell curve for ability to stay awake. There also appears that there is a bell curve for stupidity.

Also different regions have different acceptable levels of maximum blood alcohol in order to operate machinery.

[51] Banks S, Dinger DF, Behavioral and Physiological Consequences of Sleep Restriction. Journal of Clinical Sleep Medicine, August 2007; 3(5):519-528

[52] Crew Resource Management Manual. Copyright, Moncton Flight College.

[53] Air operators monitor the flight time, flight duty time and rest periods of each flight crew member. These include: a limit of 300 hours work in 90 days; a maximum of 14 hours in 24 hours: a limit of 8 hours in 24 hours for single pilot flights and a limit of 40 hours in 7 days. There are also compulsory rest periods.

Rules for truckers include 70 hours maximum a week; maximum of 13 hours a day in Canada and 11 hours a day in the U.S., after which they must take at least 10 hours rest.

[54] Crew Resource Management Manual, Copyright Moncton Flight College.

[55] I was ten when I recalled a sales man boasting to my father how by dint of will, he could drive home after being awake for twenty four hours. This myth endures. See footnote 50 above.

[56] Gadois, C. Women on night shift: interdependence of sleep and off-the-job activities. In Reinberg A, Vieux, N and Andlauser, P(eds). Night and shift work: biological and social aspects. Oxford: Pergamon Press, 1981, pp. 223-227. This study showed that married female shift workers sleep about nine hours per week less than their unmarried female colleagues.

[57] http://www.circadian.org/vital.html (The material posted on this website is based upon work supported by the National Science Foundation and the National Institutes of Health.)

[58] Conroy et al., Daily Rhythms of Cerebral Blood Flow Velocity. Journal of Circadian Rhythms 2005 3:3

[59] Lamond N, et al., Adaptation of Performance during a Week of Simulated Night Work. Ergonomics. 2004 Feb 5 :47(2):154-65.

Fifteen young individuals participated in two counterbalanced conditions which required them to (1) "work" seven consecutive 9-hour night shifts, and (2) consume alcoholic beverage at hourly intervals until their blood alcohol concentration (BAC) reached 0.10%. In each condition, performance was measured at hourly intervals using a 10-minute psychomotor vigilance test (VAT). Analysis indicated that as BAC increased, performance impairment significantly increased. Similarly, response time significantly increased during the first six night-shifts, and lapse frequency significantly increased during the first two shifts. Equating the two conditions indicated that the first stimulated night shift was associated with the greatest degree of performance impairment. In general, the impairment at the end of this shift was greater than observed at a BAC of 0.05%. For the final four hours, the performance decrements generally did not exceed those observed at a BAC of 0.05%. This suggests that during a week of consecutive night shifts, adaptation of performance occurs.

[60] GOOMER From "Intern" by Doctor X, Harper Row, New York, 1965. The "goomer" attitude is an aggressive form of labeling. My goomer attitude even extended to some who did not present at my emergency department. One New Year's Eve we had been in the Trauma Room all night with accidents, when we received a call that two ambulances were dispatched for another accident. There were four seriously injured. We scrambled to make beds available in the Trauma Room for them. About twenty minutes later we received word that none had survived. I was so relieved I was almost happy with the news of their death. I had forgotten John Dunne's "No man is an island en- tire of itself; every man is a piece of the continent." Those killed would be lost by their friends and relatives. Maybe those dead were relatives or friends of mine? I blushed at my relief, but realized that sleep starvation is a cheap drunk which can capsize diligence to apathy and tragedy to relief.

[61] Chief Dan George. My Heart Soars. Hancock House Publishers, Saanichton, B.C. Canada. 1974

[62] Ely J.W. et al. See above.

[63] Ely J.W. et al. See above.

[64] Mawardi BH, Satisfaction, Dissatisfactions, and Causes of Stress in

Medical Practice. JAMA, April 6, 1979-Vol 241,(14):148-36.

[65] The Medical Post, December 2, 2003 page 57.

[66] John Donne differentiated two attitudes to time, in the first stanza of "The Rising Sun."

"Busy old fool, unruly sun,
Why dost thou thus,
Through windows, and through curtains call on us?
Must to thy motions lovers' seasons run?
Saucy pedantic wretch, go chide
Late school-boys, and sour prendices,
Go tell court-huntsmen, that the King will ride,
Call country ants to harvest offices:
Love, all alike, no season knows, nor clime,
Nor hours, days, months, which are the rags of time."

Even in the 16th century, the time bullied: herded students along, goaded slow apprentices to be more productive, warned the king's sycophants that the king is about to go hunting, and ordered the harvest to be gathered. Are doctors to be also bullied by time or can the practice of medicine like love?, "…no season knows, nor clime,

Nor hours, days, months, which are the rags of time."

I am indebted to Mr. Lauchlin MacDowell, owner of "Rags of Time," for introducing me to this poem.

[67] Kussmaul's respirations are deep and regular usually due to metabolic acidosis.

[68] Ely, John W. (see above).

[69] An in-depth account of this disaster is related at: http://www.panamair.org/accidents/victor.htm

[70] Dorothy and Orville Messenger, "Borrowed Time." This parable demonstrates the alchemy of patience.

[71] This poise of Dr. Messenger exemplifies Ms. Wallie Simieritsch's counsel, "approach the patient with curiosity."

[72] Ely, John W., Perceived Causes of Family Physicians' Errors (see above). Note the emphatic denial. For now, I would like to add Newman's epiphany on emphasis: "to say that something must be, is to admit that it may not be." Further defence of hypotheses is addressed

in Chapter 12, "Listening for the Whisper of Doubt Within."

[73] This is the author's variation on Huxley's quotation in the Introduction.

[74] Christensen J.F. *et al*, see above. Also 9% of physicians in the Ely group blamed their wrong decisions on pride in their abilities. This coincides with Pirsig, "if you have a high evaluation of yourself then your ability to recognize new facts is weakened."(from Zen and the Art of Motorcycle Maintenance).

[75] A more subtle, but just as treacherous, emotion is the genuine concern that no consultant should be woken, even the most helpful and willing of consultants. A colleague expressed, "I would prefer trauma to come in, than have to get a consultant out of bed to come in." This often reflects as much some consultants' reluctance to leave their lair, as the reluctance of many requesting physicians to trouble them. When both these characteristics collide, disaster can happen as with the patient who had the G.I. bleed.

[76] Lewis C.S. Mere Christianity, Harper Collins

[77] Lewis C.S.(see above).

[78] Lewis C.S. "Mere Christianity", Harper Collins. Lewis continues, "Do not imagine that if you meet a really humble man, he will be what most people call humble nowadays. He is of the sort of greasy, smarmy person who is always telling you that of course he is nobody."

[79] In the medical arena, reptilian activities are feebly countered (and often accepted) in comparison with the aviation industry. In the cockpit, there is a level playing field, where junior officers are empowered to challenge the hypotheses and or hazardous attitudes of their superiors. I know of a physician who ridiculed a patient's suggestion of self-diagnosis by lying on the examining table and saying, "so you're the doctor now."

[80] This balanced epigram is by Andre Comte-Sponville's, "A Small Treatise on the Great Virtues." Pub, Henry Holt & Co. New York 1996.

[81] A Professional Pilot's Crew Resource Management Manual, Moncton Flight College. "Situational awareness refers to one's ability to accurately perceive what is going on in the cockpit and outside the aircraft. True situational awareness is an individual's accurate percep-

tion of reality."

[82] Grasha Anthony at "The Second Halifax Symposium on Health-care Error" 2002

[83] Christensen JF. Et al, see above.

[84] Quoted in Dr. Jack McCue's article, "The Effects of Stress on Physicians and their Medical Practice" New Eng J. Med 1982 Feb 25: 458-463.The term was attributed to Fox R. C. in an address delivered to faculty and residents at Cleveland Metropolitan General Hospital, May 5, 1981.

[85] A Professional Pilot's Crew Resource Management Manual, Moncton Flight College. The same source claims that, "chronic stress can affect the pilot's ability to deal with complex tasks: pilots become preoccupied with a single task, and forget or omit procedural steps; they also have a greater tendency to misconceptions, and misread gauges."

[86] Perceived Causes of Family Physicians' Errors, by John W. Ely, and others. See above.

[87] Canadian Medical Association Survey 2003.About 8,000 physicians were polled. How many of those who did not reply to the questionnaire were also suffering burnout?

[88] Deckard G, Hicks L, Hamory B.The Occurrence and Distribution of Burnout among Infectious Diseases Physicians. J. Infect Dis 1992; 165-224.

[89] Mawardi, BH. Medical Educational Meeting of the American Medical Association, 1973. Quoted in JAMA. April 6, 1979-Vol 241, No.14 p.1485

[90] Modlin HC, Montes A. Narcotic Addiction in Physicians. Am J Psychiatry. 1964; 121:358-65.(In this study, physicians were compared to a second group which were not physicians).

[91] Vaillant GE, Sobowale NC, McArthur C. Some Psychologic Vulnerabilities of Physicians. N Engl J Med. 1972; 287:272-5.

[92] Rose KD, Rosow I. Physicians Who Kill Themselves. Arch Gen Psychiatry. 1973; 29:800-5.

[93] Mawardi BH, JAMA, April 6, 197-vol 241, no14. Quoted in Medical Tribune April 5, 1967, p.15.

[94] Ross M. Suicide among Physicians. Psychiatry Med. 1971; 2: 189-98.

[95] Thomas RB, Luber SA, Smith JA. A Survey of Alcohol and Drug use in Medical Students. Dis Nerv Syst. 1977; 38:41-3.

[96] Modin HC, Montes A. See above.

[97] Valko RJ, Clayton PJ. Depression in the Internship. Dis Nerv Syst. 1075; 36:26-9.

[98] Ford CV. The Emotional Distress of Interns and Residents. Presented at the 134 American Psychiatric Association annual meeting New Orleans, La. May 1981.

[99] Valko RJ, *et al* see above.

[100] In the Deckard study above, 44% of physicians suffered emotional exhaustion; 40% Depersonalization and 8% reported feelings of low personal achievement.

[101] Pirsig, Robert. See above

[102] Authors have pointed to the metaphor of the wounded healer as highly relevant to nursing. From Cohen-Katz J, Wiley SD, Capuano T, Baker DM, Shapiro S. The Effects of Mindfulness-based Stress Reduction on Nurse Stress and Burnout: Holist Nurs Pract 2004; 18(6): 302-308. These authors reference: Jackson C. Healing Ourselves, Healing Others. Holist Nurs Pract. 2004; 18(1): 67-81; and Conti-O'Hare M.T The Nurse as Wounded Healer: From Trauma to Transcendence. Boston: Jones & Barlett Publishers; 2002.

[103] McCue J., "The Effects of Stress on Physicians and their Medical Practice" New Eng J. Med 1982 Feb 25: 458-463

[104] Onen Sertoz, *et al*, Prog Neuropsychopharmacol Biol Psychiatry, 2008 Aug: 32(6):1459-65, pub 2008 May 8. This difference was statistically significant ($p=0.005$). They also found that sBDTF levels correlated negatively with emotional exhaustion, depersonalization and correlated positively with competence sub-scales of burnout inventory.

[105] Most of the effects of burnout are expressions of the reptilian brain.

Exhaustion:

-Apathetic, complacent, taking short-cuts, for example, laying in ambush for symptoms which are the least strenuous for us to pursue.

-Distracted, jumpy, inattentive to the task at hand.

-Serving the convenient, shirking the inconvenient.

–Haste: Pressing: Impulsivity, Fretting about time.

-Making assumptions, lunging, guessing.

-Irritability-we lack a sense of humor or perspective.

-Reacting as opposed to reflection and responding.

Depersonalisation:

-Labeling (disliking) others and processes.

-Egoism, to prioritize one's agenda, one's self-esteem more than the patient's well-being.

[106] From Easter 1916, by W. B. Yeats

[107] Wright, S. Feel the Burn. Nursing Standard, 17(25), 25, 2003.

[108] Gautam Mamta. Iron doc: Practical Stress Management Tools for Physicians. Book Coach Press, Ottawa 2004

[109] Groves, James E., MD. "Taking Care of the Hateful Patient, The New England Journal of Medicine. Vol 298, No.16, pp.883-887. He describes four stereotypes: "dependent clingers; entitled demanders; manipulative help-rejecters and self-destructive deniers." He also de- scribes a physician's negative reaction to each group: "clingers evoke aversion; demanders evoke a wish to counterattack; help-rejecters evoke depression; self-destructive deniers evoke feelings of malice."

[110] Asler G, Helplessness in the Helpers. Br J Med Psychol 45:315-326, 1972

[111] CMAJ. 1998;195:525-8.

[112] Quoted in Gautam Mamta. See above

[113] Canadian Medical Association Survey, 2003.

[114] Arch Intern Med. 2000; 160:3209-14.

[115] Here are two such links:
http://www.mindtools.com/stress/Brn/BurnoutSelfTest.htm
http://psychologytoday.psychtests.com/tests/burnout2_r_access.html

[116] Gautam Mamta. See above

[117]
For example: Canadian Medical Association for Physician Health and Well-being: www.cma.ca. In the United States, AMA Physician Health Program at 312-464-5066. In Canada and the United States, there are corresponding provincial and state programs to treat physi-

cians who are not coping with their stresses.

[118] The twenty tips of Dr. Mamta Gautam are: Take care of yourself first; Get your own family doctor; Time management; Set priorities; Anticipate and prepare situations; Consider and use options; Learn to say NO; Add fun to work; Plan for transition times; Don't take your work home; Take regular time off; Use support systems; Share your stories; Remember the 90:10 Rule; Set realistic expectations; Learn a relaxation technique; Laugh more often; Take solo time; Plan your finances; Let go of the guilt.

[119] Frankl V. See above.

[120] Cohen-Katz J, Wiley SD, Capuano T, Baker DM, Shapiro S. The Effects of Mindfulness-based Stress Reduction on Nurse Stress and Burnout, Part 11: Holist Nurs Pract 2005; 19(1):26-35

Cohen-Katz J, Wiley SD, Capuano T, Baker DM, Shapiro S. The Effects of Mindfulness-based Stress Reduction on Nurse Stress and Burnout, Part 111: Holist Nurs Pract 2005; 19(2):78-86

[121] Dr. Allison Dysart expands this transposition as "a type of transcendence."

[122] Frankl V., p.94. See above.

[123] This transposition for objectivity also enables one to follow Frankl's Categorical Imperative: "Live as if you were living already for the second time and as if you had acted the first time as wrongly as you are about to act now!"

[124] Thich Nhat Hanh, monk, author, and peace activist. Author of "Be Free where you are." (Paralax Press P.O. 7355 Berkeley, California 94707) which is an account of Thich Nhat Hanh's talk with prisoners at Maryland Correctional Institute at Hangerstown in 1999. Some quotes from this talk: "Everyone walks on the earth, some walk like slaves, with no freedom at all... They are sucked in by the future or by the past and they are not capable of living in the here and now where life is available....You, (the prisoner), can scrub the floors as a free person or as a slave..." (the prisoner), my inclusion.

[125] Through the support of Ed Lamond, proprietor of "The Attic Owl," I ordered twenty copies of Frankl's "Man's Search for Meaning" and had the public read it. At a later public discussion of the book, this exchange took place.

[126] Clever L., A checklist for making good choices in trying — or tranquil — times. West J Med. 2001;174: 41-43

[127] Sartre, Jean Paul. The Reprieve.

[128] Richard Lovelace (1618-1658) was imprisoned after he petitioned the English Parliament in King Charles account. He was committed to the Gatehouse in Westminster, where he composed "To Althea, from Prison."

[129] Aiken, L.H., Clarke, S.P., Sloane, D.M., Sochalski, J.A., Busse, R., Clarke, H., *et al.* Nurses' Reports on Hospital Care in Five Countries. Health Affairs, 20(3), 43-53:2001. Nurses also face extraordinary stresses at work: extended work hours, giving intense emotional support in the face of patients' suffering, having little control in physician-controlled work environments and dealing daily with pain, loss and traumatic illness events... the problem of nursing shortages and their consequences have exacerbated the situation.

[130] Kabat-Zinn J. Full Catastrophe Living: Using the Wisdom of Your Body and Mind to Face Stress, Pain, and Illness. New York: Delta; 1990.

[131] Cohen-Katz J, Wiley SD, Capuano T, Baker DM, Shapiro S. The Effects of Mindfulness-based Stress Reduction on Nurse Stress and Burnout. Holist Nurs Pract. 2004;18(6): 302-308. Part I reported on the rationale for offering MBSR to nurses and the process of developing and implementing a program within the LVHHN system. A similar course was taken by medical and premedical students with similar encouraging results. Shapiro Shauma, L, Schwartz Gary E., Bonner Ginny. Effects of Mindfulness-based Stress Reduction on Medical and Premedical Students. Journal of Behavioral Medicine, Vol. 21, No. 6. 1998.

[132] Cohen-Katz J, Wiley SD, Capuano T, Baker DM, Shapiro S. The Effects of Mindfulness-based Stress Reduction on Nurse Stress and Burnout, Part II: Holist Nurs Pract 2005; 19(1):26-35

[133] Cohen-Katz J, Wiley SD, Capuano T, Baker DM, Shapiro S. The Effects of Mindfulness-based Stress Reduction on Nurse Stress and Burnout, Part III: Holist Nurs Pract 2005; 19(2):78-86

[134] Kabat-Zinn J. Full Catastrophe Living; Using the Wisdom of Your body and Mind to Face, Stress, Pain, and Illness." New York; Delta; 1990

[135] For more on the techniques of Mindfulness see "Full Catastro-

phe Living; Using the Wisdom of Your body and Mind to Face, Stress, Pain, and Illness." Kabat-Zinn J. New York; Delta; 1990

[136] In Zen and the Art of Motorcycle Maintenance, Pirsig describes how monks could find stamina by looking to the action and not to the fruits of the action. He also describes how he fatigued when he looked to the finish and not to the task at hand, when one gets ahead of oneself. "Phaedrus wrote a letter from India about a pilgrimage to Holy Kailash, the source of the Ganges and the abode of Shiva, high in the Himalayas, in the company of a holy man and his adherents.

"He never reached the mountain. After the third day he gave up, exhausted and the pilgrimage went on without him. He said he had the physical strength but that physical strength wasn't enough. He had the intellectual motivation but that wasn't enough either. He didn't think he had been arrogant but thought that he was undertaking the pilgrimage to broaden his experience, to gain understanding for himself. He was trying to use the mountain for his own purposes and the pilgrimage too. He regarded himself as the fixed entity, not the pilgrimage or the mountain, and thus wasn't ready for it. He speculated that the other pilgrims, the ones who reached the mountain, probably sensed the holiness of the mountain so intensely that each footstep was an act of devotion, an act of submission to this holiness. The holiness of the mountain infused into their own spirits enabled them to endure far more than anything he, with his greater physical strength, could take.

"To the untrained eye ego-climbing and selfless climbing may appear identical. Both kinds of climbers place one foot in front of the other. Both breathe in and out at the same rate. Both stop when tired. Both go forward when rested. But what a difference! The ego-climber is like an instrument that's out of adjustment. He puts a foot down an instant too soon or too late. He's likely to miss a beautiful passage of sunlight through the trees. He goes on when the sloppiness of his step shows that he is tired. He rests at odd times. He looks up the trail trying to see what's ahead because he just looked a second before. He goes too fast or too slow for the conditions and when he talks, his talk is forever about somewhere else, something else. He's here but he's not here. He rejects the here, is unhappy with it, wants to be further up the trail but when he gets there will be just as unhappy because it will be "here." What he is looking for, what he wants, is all around him, but he doesn't want that because it is all around him. Every step's an effort, both physically and spiritually, because he imagines his goal to be external and distant."

[137] Diener, E., Sandvik, E., and Pavot W. Happiness is the frequency, not the intensity, of positive versus negative affect. In "Subjective Well-Being: an interdisciplinary perspective." Ed. By Fritz Strack, Michael Argyle and Norbert Schwarz. Pergamon Press, Oxford 1991.

[138] Attributed to Henry J, Henry L. Caring from the inside out: strategies to enhance nurse retention and patient satisfaction. Nurs Leader. 2004; 2(1): 28-32.This attribution was quoted in Cohen-Katz J, article, Footnote 43 above.

[139] Dr. Pat Croskerry claimed this at "Risky Business Road Show," Montreal. December 2009.

[140] Bergson, Henri, "Introduction to Metaphysics."

[141] Bergson, Henri, "Introduction to Metaphysics."

[142] Sherlock Holmes advised, 'theories should fit the data, not data fit the theories."

[143] Dr. Allison Dysart wrote to me on this point, "We, in medicine, tend to treat diagnostic categories as if they were real, more real than the story that the patient may tell. It's like we're Platonists, with our di- agnostic categories as the Forms (real) and nature (or patients and their symptoms and their physical findings) as a poor imitation."

[144] The question might be asked, "how can we differentiate Pirsig's peace of mind from premature closure and complacency?" It may be difficult, but some clues may present by asking a few questions: Would I like to be tended as I am tending now? Is this way more convenient than another? Am I more irritable now? Am I labeling this patient or others involved? Do I command the reserve to welcome egregious, or challenging data?

[145] I am indebted to Arthur Koestler's "The Ghost in the Machine", Hutchinson & Co, London 1967. Koestler had adopted Garsang's diagram (explaining the process of evolution by paedomorphosis) to explain undoing and redoing in the evolution of ideas.

[146] Frankl V. 175.

[147] Frankl V. used the word, "responsibleness" instead of responsibility.

[148] Vaideanu, D, Fraser K, Deady JP. "Just another Corneal Abrasion?" Lancet 2002; 359: 1916.

[149] Myosis should read mydriasis. I thank Dr. Gilles Cormier for this correction.

[150] Dr. P. Croskerry, prizes this question. He recommends that as each graduating physician is given their certificate, they should also receive a medallion with the question, "What else could this be?"

[151] Pathgnomonic is sign or symptom that is so characteristic of a disease that it makes the diagnosis.

[152] Dr. Croskerry also co-authored the highly acclaimed "Patient Safety in Emergency Medicine" 2009

[153] Croskerry P., Avoiding Pitfalls in the Emergency Room. The Canadian Journal of CME April 1996.

[154] The Way of Life by Lao Tzu: trans. by R. B. Blakney, New American Library, New York, 1955.

[155] Philip Sydney's over 400 years ago prayed for deliverance from the "self-chosen snare" of desire. (Sentiments echoed by Pasteur: "The greatest disorder of the mind is to allow the will to direct belief)."

"Thou blind Man's mark, thou fool's self-chosen snare, Fond fancy scum, and dregs of scattered thought:

Band of all evils, cradle of causeless care;
Thou web of will, whose end is never wrought;
Desire, desire! I have too dearly bought,
With price of mangled mind, thy worthless ware;
Too long, too long, asleep thou hast me brought,
Who should my mind to higher things prepare.
But yet in vain thou hast my ruin sought;
In vain thou madest me to vain things aspire;
In vain thou kindlest all thy smoky fire;
For virtue hath this lesson better taught-
Within myself to seek my only hire,
Desiring naught but how to kill desire."

(Mark means target and Band means swaddling band).

[156] John W. Ely and others, for example, see No. 6 of the verbatim accounts: "… And I'm really angry now. And by this time I'm not listening."

[157] Plat. F. W. & McMath J. C.; Clinical Hypocompetence: the interview. Ann Intern med. 1979 Dec; 91 (6): 898-902.

[158] The other four shortcomings were:

A. Not asking for basic symptoms, but being content with secondary information such as lab data told to the patient and the interpretations of other doctors as relayed by the patient.

B. Neglecting to learn much about the patient's life-style.

C. Not taking into account "the sort of person" the patient is.

D. The failure of the doctor to give emotional support and healing to the patient during the interview.

[159] The Pilot's Crew Resource Management Manual describes closed and open questions depending on the information required. Closed questions are useful for getting specific information quickly. Closed questions, however, restrict the range of possible answers and can make the other feel that they are being interrogated. By comparison, open-ended or probing questions allow the person more freedom of response.

[160] The headings were titled: Active listening, Active listening is, Active listening is not, The art of effective listening, and Listen to more than the words.

[161] Stated in Crew Resource Management Manual, Copyright Moncton Flight College.

[162] By comparison, his waiting room chairs were commodious.

[163] Crew Resource Management Manual copyright, Moncton Flight   College

[164] This is easier if one's self-agenda is non-existent. The following formulae depict this:

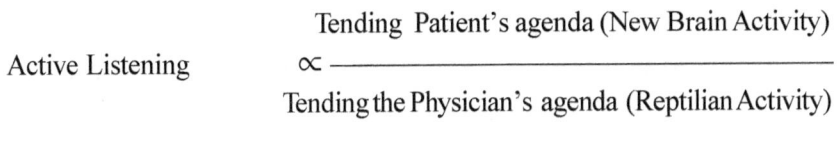

$$\text{Active Listening} \quad \propto \quad \frac{\text{Tending Patient's agenda (New Brain Activity)}}{\text{Tending the Physician's agenda (Reptilian Activity)}}$$

$$\text{Or ... Active Listening} \quad \propto \quad \frac{\text{Tending Patient's agenda}}{\text{Hurry} + \text{Fatigue} + \text{Stress} + \text{Egoism}}$$

[165] Medawar, PB. "Advice to a Young Scientist" Harper and Row,1979 Medawar's work on graft rejection and the discovery of acquired immune tolerance was fundamental to the practice of tissue and organ transplants. Medawar's comment is like the debater's tactic, when an ar- gument is weak, shout like hell.

[166] Chisholm C, Croskerry P.: A Case Study in Error: the Use of the Portfolio Entry. Academic Emergency Medicine 2004;11: 388-392. It is remarkable when we are called aside by a colleague about a case we have treated: we often know what they are going to tell us, a different diag- nosis, a different treatment or a preventable complication. Doubt dis- missed is readily recalled. Success, however, is not as easily recalled.

[167] Chuang Tzu describes this inactivity as Nothingness in "The Lost Pearl."

"The Yellow Emperor went wandering
To the North of the Red Water
To the Kwan Lun mountains. He looked around
Over the edge of the world. On the way home
He lost his night-coloured pearl.
He sent Science to seek his pearl, and got nothing.
He sent Analysis to look for his pearl, and got nothing.
He sent Logic to seek his pearl, and got nothing.
Then he asked Nothingness, and Nothingness had it!

"The Yellow Emperor said:

"Strange, indeed: Nothingness
Who was not sent
Who did not work to find it
Had the night-coloured pearl!"
(Recreated by Thomas Merton:The Way of Chuang Tzu. Penguin Books, Canada 1969)

[168] The aviation industry warns about quitting times decisions: they call it "go-home-itis." Skiing accidents are more common when the skiers race to catch the last lift up the mountain.

[169] In the Buddhist tradition also, attachment is the obstacle to enlightenment.

[170] The author's classification of doubts.

[171] Two anesthetist friends of mine were going for a plane ride. One, observing his colleague carefully inspect his plane on the outside before entering his plane, asked him, "Why are you checking the plane? You never inspect your anaesthetic machine before giving an anaesthetic." His colleague, the pilot replies, "the difference is, it is my f.......life."

[172] The CRM manual states that true situational awareness is an individual's accurate perception of reality. The "Theory of the Situation" is what one assumes to be true for a specific period of time. If a discrepancy exists between the individual's Theory of the Situation and the Reality of the Situation, a loss of situational awareness occurs and an error chain could begin.

[173] In its Crew Resource Management Manual, the authors continue: "As humans we are aware of many cues from our surroundings for which we cannot always identify the origin. These cues are very real. Don't ignore them, even when they only manifest themselves in a feeling of uneasiness."

[174] Some physicians change the tone and pitch of their voice from high register for a poor patient to a lower register for a litigation lawyer. This is another example of Frankl's claim that our freedom to respond is inalienable.

[175] Major Ralph H. Classic Descriptions of Diseases. Thomas Boots, Springfield, Illinois. 1945.

[176] Some might claim that there are other standards to judge the best physicians, like compassion or availability.

[177] To know one's self is to know one's reptilian brain.

[178] Marcus Aurelius gives us hope, "Practise thyself even in things which thou despairest of accomplishing. For even the left hand, which is ineffectual for all other things for want of practice, holds the bridle more vigorously than the right hand; for it has been practised in this."

[179] It is essential to give feedback when another has made a mistake. This feedback is better received when given in private. Sometimes when the feedback is received, ownership of the mistake is not admit-

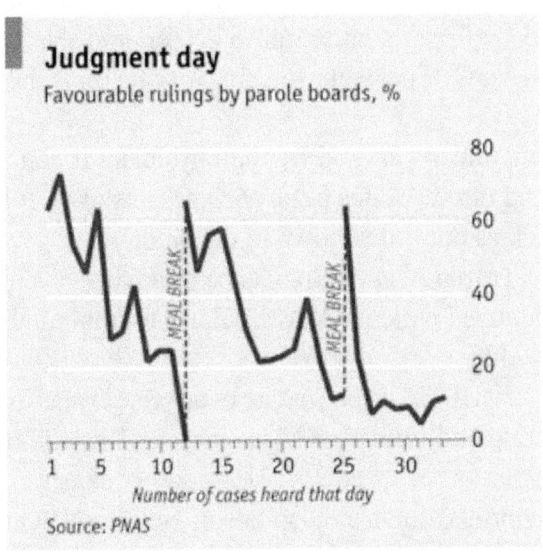

Judgment day
Favourable rulings by parole boards, %

Number of cases heard that day

Source: PNAS

ted. For example, I recall seeing a patient who presented with pain in the right shoulder. His family physician had referred him to an orthopedic surgeon, who had injected the shoulder twice with Cortisone without relief. Upon examining the patient, I found that movement of his shoulder had no effect on the pain; the pain was referred. Chest X-Ray revealed a large opacity in the right upper lobe, a Pancoast's tumor. When I related this to the orthopedic surgeon, he replied, "I always thought that there was something funny about that chap."

[180] The Economist Apr 14 2011: Court rulings depend partly on when the judge last had a snack. The article cites a paper in the *Proceedings of the National Academy of Sciences* describing how Shai Danziger of Ben-Gurion University of the Negev and his colleagues followed eight Israeli judges for ten months as they ruled on over 1,000 appli-

cations made by prisoners to parole boards.

The following graph shows how favorable rulings decreased just before breaks for meals and improved after the meals. Even after controlling for recidivism and rehabilitation programs, the meal-related pattern remained.

Resonant of Pope's couplet, written 1712:

"The hungry judges soon the sentence sign,

And wretches hang that jurymen may dine;"

[181] From Introduction to Metaphysics by Henri Bergson

[182] Inspired by Pirsig's epigraph to - "Zen and the Art of Motorcycle Maintenance," "The cycle you are working on is the cycle called yourself."

[183] Iatrogenic means caused by the physician. It can apply to adverse events and often applies to physicians' mistakes. It is frequently used by physicians but little known to the public.

[184] Brennan Troyen A. *et al.*, Incidence of adverse events and negligence in hospitalized patients. New England Journal of Medicine, Feb 1991; 324: 370-376.

[185] Leape Lucian L. *et al.*, The nature of adverse events in hospitalized patients. New England Journal of Medicine, Feb 1991; 324: 377-383.

[186] These doctors reviewed 30,121 randomly selected charts from 51 acute care, non-psychiatric hospitals in New York State in 1984 to determine the incidence of adverse events and negligence in hospitalized patients. They defined adverse events as an injury that was caused by medical management (rather than the underlying disease) and that prolonged the hospitalization, and that produced a disability at the time of discharge. The physicians identified 1278 adverse events, 972 with no negligence and 306 with negligence. They defined negligence as care that fell below the standard expected of physicians in their community. They compared these results with the California Medical Association Medical Insurance Feasibility Study, (Mills DH. West J Med 1978 Apr; 128(4): 360-365) another large scale effort to estimate the incidence of iatrogenic injury and substandard care. The Californian rate of adverse events was 4.6%, 26% higher than the Harvard Study estimate of 3.7%. The California study rate revealed a negligence rate of 0.8%, 20% lower than the Harvard Study.

[187] The authors wrote: "We could not measure all negligent acts, and made no attempt to, but measured only those that led to injury. Thus, our figures reflect not the amount of negligence, but only its consequences….(However) the judgments of physicians that an adverse event led to death also require a note of caution…… some patients may have requested and received limited care, even though the fact was not documented in the medical record.

[188] Thomas EJ, Studdert DM, Burstin HR, Orav EJ, Zeena T, Williams EJ, Howard KM, Weiler PC, Brennan TA. Incidence and types of adverse events and negligent care in Utah and Colorado. Med Care 2000 Mar; 38(3): 261-71

[189] The Institute of Medicine on page 31 of its "To Err Is Human" writes that based on the results of the New York study, "the number of deaths due to medical error may be as high as 98,000." In 20 years, the number of deaths due to medical error may be between one and two million. Intuitively as a doctor, I have doubted these numbers, yet when I tell people that I am writing a book on medical error, usually I am related a case of misdiagnosis of either themselves or a relative.

[190] Maybe concurrence of two reviewers is not a high threshold.

[191] Steel, Knight; Gertman, Paul M.; Crescenzi, Caroline , et al. Iatrogenic Illness on a General Medical Service at a University Hospital. N Engl J Med. 304: 638-642, 1981.

[192] Andrews, Lori B.; Stocking, Carol; Krizek, Thomas, et al.,An Alternative Strategy for Studying Adverse Events in Medical Care. Lancet.349: 309-313, 1997.

[193] Clarke JR, Spejewski B, Gertner AS, et al.,An objective analysis of process errors in trauma resuscitations. Acad Emerg Med. 2000; 7: 1303-1310.

[194] Wilson et al. The quality of Australian health care study. Med J Aust 1995; 163: 458-71.

[195] Davies P, et al. Acknowledgment of "no fault" medical injury: review of patients' hospital records in New Zealand. BMJ 2003;326:79-80.

[196] Baker Gr et al. The Canadian adverse events study: the incidence of adverse events among hospital patients in Canada. CMAJ 2004; 170:1678-86.

[197] "Committee on Quality of Health Care in America; Institute of

Medicine, National Academy Press, Washington D.C. 2001.

[198] "To Err is Human," "Committee on Quality of Health Care in America; Institute of Medicine, National Academy Press, Washington D.C. 2001.

[199] This was one physician recounting another's mistake, not his own.

[200] I am indebted to Dr. Ivan Cohen, of Mount Allison University for this suggestion.

[201] http://www.newyorker.com/reporting/2007/01/29/070129fa_fact_ groopman

ABOUT THE AUTHOR

John Mary Meagher graduated in medicine from the National University of Ireland, Dublin and has worked for forty years as a family physician and emergency room physician. The Theorem of Attribution, The NewMind Response™ and "Medicine, Mistakes and the Reptilian Brain" is the product of eleven years research. His thesis- novel called "A Bluebell in a Quarry" and poems and essays have been previously published. Meagher lives with his wife, Bernadette, in Moncton, Canada. They have five children and six grandchildren.

The author welcomes readers to share suggestions, experiences and critiques related to this topic at the following domain: www.fewererrors.com. Dr. Meagher can be reached for seminars and speaking engagements at the same domain.

---

[i] From Introduction to Metaphysics by Henri Bergson
[ii] Inspired by Pirsig's epigraph to "Zen and the Art of Motorcycle Maintenance," "The cycle you are working on is the cycle called yourself."

www.ingramcontent.com/pod-product-compliance
Lightning Source LLC
Chambersburg PA
CBHW051504170526
45166CB00001B/386